Changing Nursing Practice

Changing Nursing Practice

SECOND EDITION

Edited by

Stephen G Wright, RGN, RCNT, Dip N, RNT, DANS, MSc (Nursing), FRCN, MHSM, MBE

Director of The European Nursing Development Agency Ltd (TENDA),
Cumbria, UK
Visiting Professor, School of Nursing, University of Southampton, UK

A member of the Hodder Headline Group
LONDON • SYDNEY • AUCKLAND

First edition published 1989
Second edition published in Great Britain 1998 by
Arnold, a member of the Hodder Headline Group,
338 Euston Road, London NW1 3BH
http://www.arnoldpublishers.com

British Library Cataloguing in Publication Data
A catalogue record for this book is available from the British Library

Library of Congress Cataloging-in-Publication Data
A catalog record for this book is available from the Library of Congress

ISBN 0 340 63181 3

2 3 4 5 6 7 8 9 10

Publisher: Clare Parker
Production Editor: Liz Gooster
Production Controller: Rose James
Cover designer: Julie Martin

Typeset in 9½ on 11½ Palatino and Frutiger by Phoenix Photosetting, Chatham, Kent
Printed and bound in Great Britain by JW Arrowsmith, Bristol

Nurses Can Do It

For Ian

Contents

List of contributors

Donna Davenport RGN, ENB 199
Practice Nurse, formerly Sister in Accident & Emergency

Helena Kearsley RGN, SCM, NDN, CPT
Professional Advisor District Nursing and Coordinator Macmillan
Respite at Home Scheme

Dirk Keyzer PhD, MSc, RGN
Professor of Nursing, Head of Nursing Division, School of Health
Studies, University of Bradford

Sue Pearce RGN, DNCert, CPT
Professional Advisor (District Nursing)

Lesley Surman BA, RN, RCNT, OND, RNT
Nurse Teacher, The University of Manchester

Stephen Wright RGN, RCNT, Dip N, RNT, DANS, MSc (Nursing),
FRCN, MHSM, MBE
Director of The European Nursing Development Agency Ltd (TENDA),
Cumbria and Visiting Professor, School of Nursing, University of
Southampton

Preface

Knowledge is power.

Hobbes, *Leviathan*

Every nurse has wanted at some stage to change nursing not just in the grander sphere of things but at local level, in a particular ward, unit or team. I remember my bungled efforts of the past when I assumed that, because I felt I was right, everybody would agree with me, and because I was wildly enthusiastic, everyone else would feel the same way too!

Ignorance is not bliss, it leaves you vulnerable, a pawn in the struggle for power and control which can occur when haphazard change, however well intentioned, occurs.

The light began to dawn when I was fortunate enough to attend a course in which change theory and its application were covered in depth. Then it became clear that the skills needed to change things are as complex as any other regardless of the level you are working at. I was able to take this knowledge forward and use it in my practice, in just the same way as I was familiar and skilled with the use of a blanket or a bedpan.

All the contributors to this book have gone through this experience. Becoming an effective change agent requires many complex skills to be developed. Some nurses get there after many years of (often painful) experience. However, the path is both shorter and straighter if we have early access to the information we need. This book offers such information. All the contributors, having learned the intricacies of change, often felt 'if only I had known that before'. Change theory, and how to apply it to nursing practice, is therefore the subject of this book. Knowing what to change is good, knowing how to change is better.

Stephen G. Wright
Mungrisdale, Cumbria, 1997

Acknowledgements

Extract from the song 'Good Friends' by Joni Mitchell, copyright 1985 Crazy Cow Music (BMI), reproduced with kind permission of Windswept Pacific Music Limited for UK and Eire.

I would particularly like to offer my thanks to Mrs M. McDermott and Mrs I. Hill for secretarial and other support above and beyond the call of duty.

Editor's note

The words patient, client or resident are used interchangeably to describe the recipient of care. The reader is asked to interpret whichever they feel most comfortable with. The word 'clinical' is used in the general sense, referring to any area where nurses are working directly with patients, clients or residents, in hospital or community. The word 'nurse' is used throughout the text in a general sense for simplicity, and includes nurses, midwives and health visitors.

Introduction

Sometimes change comes at you
Like a broadside accident,
There is chaos to the order,
Random things, you can't prevent.
There could be trouble around the corner,
There could be beauty down the street.

Joni Mitchell, 'Good Friends'

If you have attended a meeting of nurses recently, then the chances are that the subject of 'change' has raised its head. It is hard indeed to pick up a paper, book or journal, or to switch on a television or radio, without finding the notion that 'things are changing' not just in nursing, but in the wider world around us.

Toffler (1973) writes of

the roaring current of change, a current so powerful today that it overturns institutions, shifts our values and shrivels our roots. Change is the process by which the future invades our lives, and it is important to look at it, not merely from the grand perspectives of history, but also from the vantage point of the living, breathing individuals who experience it.

This book seeks to address itself to the last point made by Toffler, for the contributors have all functioned as change agents at clinical level and much of what we write is based upon our own rich experiences. We wish to share these with you, because all nurses are caught up in change. We cannot avoid it. Like a lumbering beast entering a neat and well-protected garden, change threatens to enter all our professional lives. If we do not learn to master this beast, to ride it, and to steer it in the direction that *we* choose, then we can expect to be trampled beneath its hooves, ignored and trodden down.

So often in the past, this has happened to nurses. Powerless, apolitical and disorganised, we are swept along with change, able only to react and not to control. Change is not only inevitable, it is accelerating, and nurses will face more and more of it in years to come. With the benefit of hindsight we can often feel that the past was a simpler time of stability or slower change, while many might argue that the changes in health services in recent years have not only been frequent but cumulative. We can often feel overwhelmed by the prospect of change, perhaps even more so when an endless steam of requests and commands pile upon us. In the past few years we have seen a major restructuring of the the health services in the UK. At the same time, nursing education has been relocated into higher education and transformed by Project 2000. Nursing Development Units, Primary Nursing, Nursing Models, Nursing Standards, Nurse Practitioners, Clinical Supervision, Clinical Audit, Patient's Charters, Clinical Grading – and more – wave after wave of changes have crashed upon nursing, some piling up simultaneously. Little wonder, then, that so many of us feel that there has never been a time when so much change is expected of us all at once. Some nurses have embraced these new ideas with skill and enthusiasm, others have felt afraid and disempowered.

In learning how to manage change, nurses can become effective change agents; however this is merely the beginning. The process of change, when set in motion, rolls on into the future as the change agent creates the 'clinical laboratory' (Infante, 1980) where others learn to accept change as a normal part of the culture. The Nursing Development Unit movement (Salvage and Wright 1995), for example, which began in the early 1980s, embodied this spirit of creating nursing, and indeed multidisciplinary, settings where 'change is a way of life'.

Producing a climate of this nature is not easy for nurses, and in many ways it runs counter to the traditional perception of a professional. The tendency for professions to be elitist, controlling their members and their clients, is alien to the process of change advocated in this book. The nurse change agent works as partner and companion with both colleagues and client turning 'the servant into the master through the use of expertise' (Wilkes, 1981). Indeed, it may be argued that one of the traditional hallmarks of professions is the use (or abuse) of their powers to resist change. There is little need for nursing to become a pillar of the establishment, there are more than enough of these. Rather, nursing can advocate a new form of professionalism. Through the acquisition of knowledge, skill, expertise or influence – some of the components of power – nurses can act not for their own self-aggrandisement or to control others, but to empower others to take control of their destinies for themselves.

Campbell (1984) has argued that such a course is immensely difficult for nurses, for it demands altruism: 'the professional gains knowledge to help, but that knowledge gives both detachment and power. It is a hard demand that the detachment should not be used for the protection of self, nor the power for the enhancement of self'. The use of such power demands not only a love of the self, but a love of others in order to give of that power to help. Such a form of 'moderated love', states Campbell, underpins the ability of the nurse to act as a change agent. In addition, being more aware of ourselves and what makes us 'tick' is part of what makes successful change agents, and we will consider this issue further in later chapters when we look at how we take care of ourselves and attend to our own needs while attending to the needs of nursing.

The call to nurses to take on the mantle of change agency is also a call to take both political and personal action. The two need not necessarily be separated; indeed the position of nurses is a challenge for us to combine or hybridise the two. Halmos (1978) tends to segregate the two as distinct and incompatible forms of change agency. The political change agent is seen as partisan and tending to deal with people as massed groups (e.g. divided by class, occupation or role). The personalist is less judgemental and focuses on dealing with individuals. The politicalist is characterised as domineering, using others to achieve their ends in Machiavellian style. The personalist works less certainly and is non-manipulative (Campbell, 1984). Nurses have the opportunity to be hybrids of these seemingly opposing poles. On the one hand we may work with individual colleagues or clients to produce awareness and assistance in change; or we might work to produce innovation in a small, local way in our own ward or team. On the other hand, we can participate in wider political movements, both inside and outside the profession and the organisations in which we work. Clinical nurses are in a position to merge the two trends, to become hybrid change agents at personal and political levels, generating change in all manner of circumstances.

This book is aimed at such nurses and those who support them, be it on wards, in nursing homes or in the community. How often are we called upon to change things. Implement the nursing process! Use a model! Change to primary nursing! Identify the 'named nurse'! These and hundreds of other issues face clinical nurses today. It is relatively easy to attend a meeting or a conference and to learn *what* a new idea is all about. A quick lecture can soon fill us with the facts on a particular subject. The problem often arises when we try to put the idea into action. We can feel shocked and disillusioned when what we perceive to be a perfectly sensible idea is greeted with disbelief, resistance and even hostility from colleagues.

It is not surprising that nurses can find it difficult to be creative or to take on board new ideas. Surrounded by multitudes of work pressures, and with their nose to the wheel and elbow to the grindstone, it is very difficult to look up and have a vision of new horizons! In addition, many nurses have not experienced progressive approaches which encourage them to learn and to develop ideas and put them into action.

Yet, as Toffler (1973) says, 'We are all in the business of change' and, if we are to manage that business well, we need to learn and practise its skills. Knowing what change is and how to take control of it can be learned, just as we can learn how to take a temperature correctly or give pills safely.

However, the opportunities to learn the skills of managing change are still relatively rare in nursing, unless we get there ourselves by dint of our own experience and intuition. Perhaps it is no accident that nurses are rarely taught to master change. The *status quo* of the social order, both inside and outside nursing, might feel a little uncomfortable at the prospect. For example, just imagine what a force for change the 600 000 nurses in the UK would represent! What would be the effects, not only on the health system, but also on society at large, if an army of skilled, assertive and aware change experts (most of whom would be women) was unleashed upon them?

However, nurses must be skilful change agents for two principal reasons. First, because nursing has the potential to contribute to the health and well-being of individuals and society as a whole. If we believe what we do is for the good of others, then we must ensure that we can better control what we do so that the recipient of our services, the patient or client, gets the best deal from us. Not everyone in health care always has the best interests of the patient at heart. As Machiavelli (1961) succinctly noted, 'the fact is that a man who wants to act virtuously in every way, necessarily comes to grief among so many who are not virtuous'. Changing and organising the health care system is like a giant game with a multitude of players. Playing the game while ignorant of its rules is doomed to failure. When nurses fail, they may fail their patients too. Second, change produces stress for us as individuals. It is even more stressful if we feel that everything around us is beyond our control. We might resent the change because it frightens us or because we do not understand, but sooner or later change gets forced upon us for good or ill. Not all change makes things better! So we must be able to understand the nature of change, not only so that we are better able to determine its course, but also so that we can protect ourselves and our patients. Many nurses are damaged humans as a result of change forced upon them throughout their lives, and not just in nursing, as Snow and Willard's (1991) study suggests, leaving them able only to react and resent.

Knowledge is power, and knowledge of change helps to give nurses the power over change. Thus empowered we are not left merely to react, but may indeed be proactive in determining the course that nursing takes. Doing this, we serve not only the interests of ourselves but the interests of those we exist to help.

References

Campbell, A.V. 1984 *Moderated love: a theology of professional care.* Society for Promoting Christian Knowledge, London.

Halmos, P. 1978 *The personal and the political: social work and political action.* Century Hutchinson, London.

Infante, M. 1980 *The clinical laboratory.* The C.V. Mosby Co., St Louis.

Machiavelli, N. 1961 *The prince* (Trans. by George Bull). Penguin, Hardmondsworth.

Salvage, J. and Wright, S.G. 1995 *Nursing development units – a force for change.* Scutari, Harrow.

Snow, C. and Willard, P. 1991 *I'm dying to take care of you.* Professional Counsellor Books, Redmond WA.

Toffler, A. 1973 *Future shock.* Pan Books, London.

Wilkes, R. 1981 *Social work with undervalued groups.* Tavistock Publications, London.

1 Change strategies: the classic models

Dirk Keyzer with Stephen Wright

It should be borne in mind that there is nothing more difficult to handle, more doubtful of success, and more dangerous to carry through than initiating changes in a state's constitution. The innovator makes enemies of all those who prospered under the old order, and only lukewarm support is forthcoming from those who would prosper under the new.

Machiavelli, *The Prince*

Change and innovation: an introduction to change theory

Whenever nurses meet to discuss the organisation and delivery of care, the issue of change is sure to be high on the agenda. Examples of the current changes taking place are numerous and include the introduction of nursing models in practice and education, and the reorganisation of the National Health Service, the expansion of the independent sector of health care, the implementation of project 2000, the spread of nurse practitioner roles and so on. Furthermore, organisations such as the United Kingdom Central Council and National Boards for Nursing, Midwifery and Health Visiting, government health departments and various professional groups spend a great deal of their time and money making policy decisions to encourage innovation and change in nursing.

Whilst change and innovation are everpresent in nursing organisations, it often appears that their chance of survival is slim (Keyzer, 1985). Research studies have isolated a host of professional, organisational, political and economic reasons why change in nursing organisations appears to be more apparent than real (Stacey *et al.*, 1970; Davies, 1980; Keyzer, 1985; White, 1986; Pearson, 1989; Black, 1991; Vaughan and Cole, 1995).

The problem facing nurses is not the inevitability of change, but the way in which the who, why, where, when and how of the process can be planned to achieve maximum benefit for individuals, groups, and society as a whole. Many attempts to implement change in nursing fail because of the unstructured approach adopted by the innovators, the lack of understanding of the nature of the change and the effect of the outcomes on the participants, or the lack of provision of resources needed to achieve the desired outcomes.

The purpose of this chapter is to explore the well documented and common strategies available to nurses seeking to implement change in practice, education and management. These changes and their practical application will be explored in detail in later chapters. Reference will be made to research studies utilising these strategies, but the more indepth examples of change in nursing will be left to the other chapters of this book. The need to select a strategy to guide practice will be stressed and deemed central to ensuring the success of the venture, to clarify the nurse's thoughts on the nature of the change and to make sure that the outcomes maintain or promote the dignity of human beings. Thus the moral and ethical aspects of change are acknowledged to be part of the problem-solving exercise of planned change.

Definition of terms

The term change can be defined as an attempt to alter or replace existing knowledge, skills, attitudes, norms and styles of individuals and groups. It is a discontinuity of the subjects' past behaviours and their perception of that discontinuity. Change in nursing practice, education and management begins with existing structures and processes the plan for revising them, proceeds to the actions to achieve the desired outcomes and the evaluation of the success in creating something new or different. The altered form embodies elements of the previous one (Hall, 1977; Beyers, 1984, Pearson, 1989).

Innovation can be defined as the introduction of new ideas, methods or devices. It refers to the material technology and the idea justifying that technology. Innovativeness describes a set of attitudes and values that are open to change. Innovation takes place in social systems over a period of time. It requires open channels of communication which permit the diffusion of new knowledge throughout the organisation (Hall, 1977; Keyzer, 1985).

The introduction of planned change can be viewed from two points of view: from the subjects' new behaviour, and as an example of innovation in the organisation. The process of planned change, therefore, involves the gathering of information on the innovation and on the nature and functioning of the organisation and its members. Thus, innovation in nursing practice includes the nurse, the resources available, the concepts and philosophies underlying the model for practice, and the way in which care is organised and delivered in the hospital and community setting.

The planning of change is a process in which the nurse takes deliberate actions to achieve the desired outcomes with the minimal use of resources. It is a problem-solving exercise in which the need for change and what needs to be changed is identified. The nurse plans the actions to achieve the desired outcomes, implements the plan, and evaluates the success of the venture. Parallels can be drawn between the framework used for the nursing process and the change process.

Strategies for change: meeting the challenge

The accelerated pace of modern life and the changes taking place within the provision of health care services demand that nurses develop their expertise in the management of change. Central to the facilities of change is the selection of strategies that are likely to achieve the desired outcomes. Just as nurses would select a framework for practice, or to design a curriculum, choosing a strategy for change helps to clarify the nurse's thoughts on the nature of the change, and to plan actions in a logical and orderly manner.

Chin and Benne (Bennis *et al.*, 1976), in their discussion on the development of change theory, define the process of selecting a strategy as the deliberate and conscious use and application of knowledge as a tool for modifying patterns and institutions of practice. It involves a clear understanding of the elements of the situation, restructuring the elements in the most advantageous way, and finding the best possible solution to the problem at hand. Thus, selecting a strategy for change requires the nurse to have problem-solving, decision-making and communication skills. As such, the selection of a strategy for, and the planning of, change is a legitimate part of the professional nurse's role.

Haffer (1986) supports the problem-solving approach to planned change and suggests that, once the need for change has been identified, the nurse must match the strategy to the person(s) involved in the change. Haffer argues that two important issues need to be considered

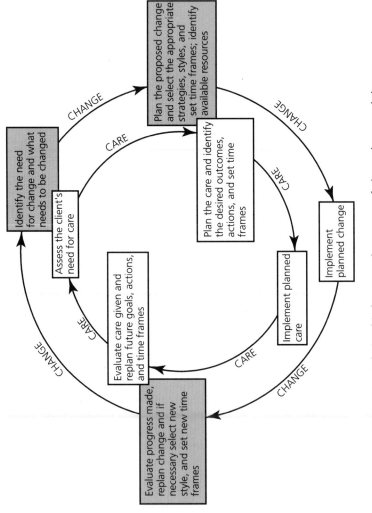

Figure 1.1 Relationship between the process of planned care and change

in selecting the appropriate strategy and to facilitate change. These considerations are:

- the strategy should focus on the appropriate change target;
- the willingness and ability of the group to change.

Towell and Harries (1979), in their discussion on innovation in patient care, also identified the need to consider how change could be perceived by experienced nurses to be some form of criticism of past practices. In particular, they refer to the dominant features of large health care institutions which include a sense of isolation from the user of the service, a traditional rigidity and pattern of hierarchical dependence, a confusion in management and lack of collaboration between professionals, and a pessimistic climate in which awareness of resource constraints and memories of past failures inhibit individual initiatives. Similar conclusions were drawn by Keyzer (1985) who further identified the effect the distribution of power and control could have on the implementation of change. As nursing research develops our awareness of the factors which promote or inhibit change in practice, so also does it highlight the need to select a strategy, or strategies, which build upon the positive and overcome the negative elements.

Sugden (1984), Beyers (1984), Keyzer (1985) and Haffer (1986) all cite Bennis *et al.* (1976) and identify three predominant change strategies. These strategies are: rational–empirical; power–coercive; and normative–re-educative. Each of these strategies is based on different assumptions about what makes people change or alter their behaviour. Each strategy is viewed by Bennis *et al.* (1976) as having potentially different degrees of success. In discussing these three individual strategies, Haffer (1986) argued that the appropriateness of each strategy depended on the situation and the individuals whose knowledge, beliefs, attitudes, values or behaviour we seek to change. Thus, the nurse's expertise in identifying the source of the demand for, and the focus of, the change is critical to the selection of appropriate strategies. This in turn implies that change theory is an essential component in basic and post basic education programmes, and that students and trained staff need exposure to role models who value and support the implementation of change in practice.

The rational–empirical strategy

A variety of strategies fall under the heading of rational–empirical. Underpinning this approach is the belief that all persons are guided by reason and that they will utilise some rational calculus of self-interest in determining needed changes of behaviour. This strategy is similar to Vinokur's model (1971) for decision-making in which it is suggested that, when faced with the possibility of choice involving risk, it is rational to select the outcomes offering the optimum value to the individual or group.

Examples of the rational–empirical strategy are the beliefs that the dissemination of research findings will change nursing practice, and that the distribution of leaflets outlining the spread of the disease AIDS will alter the population's sexual practices. Unfortunately, we do not always act on the basis of reason. We could spend much time and energy teaching a group of smokers about the danger of smoking, providing graphic detail and vast amounts of evidence of its consequences. It does not follow that they will then naturally and promptly give up smoking. Other factors are at work which affect the way we make decisions and respond to the urgings of others.

The power–coercive strategy

In the rational–empirical approach there is a basic assumption that knowledge is a major source and ingredient of power. Thus men and women of knowledge are power holders and the desirable change is achieved through the transfer of knowledge (power) to those lacking the specific knowledge in the education process (Bernstein, 1975; Bennis *et al.*, 1976; Keyzer, 1985). The power–coercive strategy emphasises a different type of power. This power is based on the use of political and economic sanctions to achieve the desired outcome and, when necessary, the use of moral power. The common assumption underlying the power–coercive strategy is that persons with less power will always comply with the plans, directives and leadership of those with greater power. This strategy is one most commonly used and associated with the historical development of nursing organisations. Examples of this strategy are to be found in everyday practice, and range from the nurse manager's right to override the decisions made by clinical staff (Towell, 1975), to the government's directives for changing the structure of the National Health Service.

Both the rational–empirical and the power–coercive strategies can be viewed as 'top-down' approaches to change. That is the need for change, the focus of the change, and the means of implementing and evaluating it, are identified by those in positions of power. The traditional attitudes of some doctors and nurses towards their patients, or teachers towards their students, provide examples of this practice. Thus, it is the doctor and the nurse who decide what the patient's needs are and how they are to be met. Similarly, it is the teacher who decides what the student needs to learn, how it will be learned, and what will constitute evidence of success or failure. Underlying these strategies is a belief in the inherent right of the power holders to exercise their power and the subject's uncritical acceptance of that right. There are many examples in both our social and professional lives to show how these strategies succeed and fail. The term 'non-compliance' is often used by nurses to describe patients who, for whatever reason, reject the nurse's perceptions of their needs for care.

Wright (1986) has argued that effective change in patient care is not only dependent on the selection of appropriate frameworks for practice, but also on the active involvement of the participants. Such a strategy is defined by Chin and Benne as normative–re-educative (Bennis *et al.*, 1976). This approach does not negate the inherent right of the power holders to define the need for change, nor to plan the actions to be taken. It seeks to reinforce these efforts to ensure the maximum benefits for all persons involved in the process.

The normative–re-educative approach

This strategy rests upon assumptions about people that contrast with those underlying the rational–empirical and power–coercive strategies. It is argued that people need to be involved in all aspects of the change process and that their actions are directed by a normative culture which involves open channels of communication in social systems and agreed norms of behaviour. In this way, changes in practice are seen to involve not only the identification of a need for change by others and the provision of information supporting that need, but also the habits and values of individuals, and the structure, roles and relationships of, and within, groups.

The normative–re-educative approach is a 'bottom-up' type of strategy the success of which depends on the individual's or group's perceptions of the need for change and its relationship to daily practices. Towell and Harries (1979) support this 'bottom-up' approach to change in nursing organisations and they provide examples of how the good ideas presented by the clinical staff can be supported to improve patient care. Similarly, Keyzer (1985), Wright (1986) and Pearson (1989), in their separate accounts of the introduction of nursing models in practice and education, have demonstrated the benefits of involving all levels of the nursing organisation in the change process. Thus, the normative–re-educative strategy is a means of bringing together the organisation's perceptions of the need for change (external needs for change) and the individual's, or group's, perception of the relationship of that change to the daily practice (internal needs for change).

Current examples of the application of the normative–re-educative strategy for change are the moves towards a more patient-centred and student-centred approach to care and education. The active involvement of the patient in identifying needs for care, selecting the actions to be taken to achieve the desired outcomes of the plan of care, and in evaluating the effectiveness of the care, is a normative–re-educative process of nursing (Keyzer, 1985; Wright, 1986; Pearson, 1989). Similarly, the devolved examination system now evident in nursing schools is believed to afford the student greater control over the content of the learning programme and the assessment of the success achieved. The use of assignments and project work as part of the 'final' examination by educational institutions seems to demonstrate how the external needs of the organisation and the internal needs of the student can be met in innovative assessment strategies.

Selecting a strategy: some questions to be asked and answered

The three strategies for change are:

- rational–empirical
- power–coercive
- normative–re-educative.

Of these, the normative–re-educative approach appears to be the one most likely to achieve real change in nursing practice. It may be necessary, however, to utilise a combination of all three strategies to achieve the desired outcome, in which case, it is important to identify which strategy has been selected to achieve the various subgoals of the proposed change (*see* Fig. 1.2).

To enable us to select the appropriate strategy, a number of questions need to be asked and answered. The following questions should help the nurse to clarify the various components of the change process and to focus attention on the specifics.

Identifying the need for change and what needs to be changed

1 *What is it that you wish to change?*
Is it a behaviour, an attitude, a skill associated with the introduction of new technology, the patient's health care practices, the student's knowledge base? A combination of all these factors?

2 *Why do you want to implement the change?*
Is it because you have been asked to implement it by others (external source), or that you yourself have identified a need for change (internal source)? Is it that both you and your colleagues (group) have perceived a need for change? Is the change being enforced by senior members of the organisation (power–coercive), by the evidence found in research reports (rational–empirical), or is it being implemented because the group themselves have initiated the actions (normative–re-educative)?

Change strategy	Leadership style
Power–Coercive	*Telling* The change agent provides information, gives orders, directs change and defines the who, what, where, when and how of change. Elements of rational–emprical strategy may be used.
Rational–Empirical	*Selling* The change agent provides information and attempts to convince the group of the need for change. Provides support for change, but is less directive than in the power–coercive approach. Elements of power–coercive and normative–re-educative strategies may be used.
Normative–Re-educative	*Participating* The change agent negotiates with the group in decision-making. Information and directions provided when asked for by the group.
	Delegating Self-directed change with minimal inputs from change agent. The individual/group may adopt the change agent role.

Figure 1.2 Relationships between change strategies and styles. After Bennis *et al.* (1976) and Hersey and Blanchard (1982)

Planning and implementing the proposed change

3 *How are you going to implement the change?*
Are you simply going to issue an order (power–coercive)? Are you going to circulate information (rational–empirical)? Are you going to discuss the need for change with the subjects, listen to their opinions, involve them in all aspects of the process and provide supportive education programmes (normative–re-educative)?

4 *Where is the change to be implemented?*
Will the change be implemented in the classroom, the ward, the patient's home, the library? A combination of these sites?

5 *When will the change be implemented?*
Do you expect the subjects to implement the change in their own time or within their working hours? Are you going to set time frames within which the subsections and the whole change are to be achieved?

6 *Which resources will be needed to implement the change?*
Have you estimated the nature and quantity of resources needed to
achieve the desired change? Does it require material, financial, manpower and educational inputs? If so, how much will it cost? Where are
these resources coming from? Have you built in manpower resources
to release staff from the clinical areas to attend the education programmes, or to reflect on the progress made? Who is going to supply
the needed resources: the organisation, or some external agency in the
form of a research grant?

7 *Who is going to implement the change?*
Are you going to implement the change yourself? Are you asking
others to change their practice, learning and/or teaching strategies,
or managerial styles? Will the change involve a group of clinical
nurses, teachers and managers? Does the change involve other
health care workers and, if so, have their needs been taken into
account? Does the change involve the patient and his or her relatives
and, if so, have their beliefs, values, norms and styles been taken
into account?

Evaluating the change and replanning the next phase of the process

8 *What effect will the change have on the role of the nurse?*
In planning the proposed change have you defined the desired outcomes? Does the proposed change alter the role of the nurse and, if so,
does it promote the role or diminish it? If the role is to be changed,
have the tasks associated with the new role been identified and differ-
entiated from those linked with the previous one? Does the new role
alter the relationships held by the nurse *vis-à-vis* the patient, other
nurse colleagues, the doctor and the manager?

9 *Which criteria are you going to use to evaluate the outcomes of the
change?*
Are you going to use quantitative or qualitative evaluation methods to
determine whether or not the desired outcomes have been achieved?
Perhaps you will need to use both of these methodologies. Which tools
are available to help you evaluate the change? Are there existing tools
in the research studies supporting the change, or ones that have been
developed by others attempting the same change? Will you have to
develop new tools for the evaluation and, if so, is there local expertise
to help you? Are you going to take the subject's perceptions of the
change achieved into account? Do you need complex computer services and programs to collate and analyse the evaluation data and, if
so, are expertise and equipment readily available to you? Will you
have to buy in expertise to help you analyse the evaluation data and, if
so, where are the resources?

10 *How are you going to communicate the results of the change?*
Are you going to write a report of the implementation of change and
the success achieved? If so, who is going to write the report? To whom
may the results be communicated? Are you going to publish articles in
the nursing journals? If so, who holds the copyright? Are you going to
report back in a study day? If so, who is going to provide the resources
for this study day? Are you going to involve the participants in the
feedback to the group and others?

Once these questions have been answered, the selection of appropriate strategies leads to the clarification of the steps to be taken in
putting the plan into action.

Putting the strategy into action

There is an increasing body of nursing knowledge (Pembrey, 1980;
Keyzer, 1985; Rafferty, 1991; Turner-Shaw and Bosanquet, 1991;
Wright, 1996) which identifies the leadership role of those in clinical
leadership positions, such as sisters and charge nurses and others who
lead clinical teams, in promoting and changing standards of care.
Whilst such roles embrace that of change agent, they cannot succeed
without the full cooperation of the staff and other health care workers.
In day-to-day practice, the clinical leader needs to communicate, coop-
erate and negotiate with doctors, managers (nurse, unit and general
managers), nurse colleagues and a host of other workers whose combined services are required to meet the goals of patient care and the
organisation.

In formulating the plan of change, the nurse must consider how that
change influences, and is influenced by, the services provided by colleagues. Beyers (1984) reinforces this need to acknowledge the recipro-
cal relationships that exist within the health service and how change in
any one part of the organisation affects the others. Thus, one of the
prime functions of the nurse is to negotiate a mutual agreement for
change within the nursing service and between the areas of the organisation. The skills of negotiation are pivotal to the success of the change
agent, as will be seen from the case studies which appear later in this
text.

In addition, for selecting a strategy, or strategies, for change, the
nurse must also select a framework which promotes the cooperation of
colleagues and other work groups. Hersey and Blanchard (1982) offer
a framework which helps the nurse to clarify thoughts about the relationships between the amount of direction and support the change
agent gives, and the degree of willingness and ability to change
expressed by the participants. This model suggests four leadership
styles the nurse can adopt to link the appropriate change strategy to
the needs of the participants. These four styles (*see* Fig. 1.2) are:

- telling
- selling
- participating
- delegating.

Telling

This style is a combination of the rational–empirical and power–coercive change strategies (*see* Fig. 1.2). An example is the decision taken by the statutory bodies to adopt nursing models and a problem-solving approach to care (GNC, 1977; UKCC, 1986). In this instance, the training institutions were provided with directives about a change in practice and education. Keyzer (1985) described how this policy decision was implemented and managed by one health authority. In this research study, the Nursing Policy Group adopted the patient-centred approach to care as official policy for all care areas. Seminars were then provided in which information was given to all nurse managers and teachers. The nursing service then set up a Nursing Process Development Group to coordinate the implementation of this policy in the clinical areas. The service, therefore, exerted only a limited control over the adoption of this change.

This approach of 'telling' the members of the group is viewed by Haffer (1986) as being most suited to those persons of low ability and willingness to change, to take responsibility for independent action, or who feel insecure and unsure of their ability to change. Individuals and groups who perceive a threat from the implementation of a particular innovation need support and education to help them through the change process. The need for supervision falls off as the individual or group gains confidence in their ability to cope with and influence the desired change.

A further example of this style is to be found in any nurse training institution where nurse teachers adopt the traditional didactic approach to teaching students. Similarly, when students first set out to review the literature on a specific nursing subject, or attempt to initiate project work as part of their course, the nurse teacher may initially adopt a 'telling' style until the student gains the experience and confidence to control the contents of the assignment. The use of broad objectives for clinical placements may also be perceived as 'telling' both clinical staff and students about the learning opportunities available in the clinical areas. In this instance, the 'telling' styles provide the safety of a framework within which the student can explore the learning opportunities available without taking on responsibilities which belong to the teacher.

Selling

This style may contain elements of the power–coercive strategy, but utilises a more rational–empirical approach to change (*see* Fig. 1.2). Keyzer (1985), Pearson (1989) and Wright (1986), in their separate approaches to implementing nursing models in practice and education, provide evidence of utilising this approach. Keyzer (1985), for example, described the use of seminars, study days and workshops to help disseminate information on, and develop nursing expertise in, problem identification, problem-solving and the implementation of the nursing process. In this study, the nurses attempting to change their mode of practice were invited to contribute to these learning programmes and were, therefore, active in 'selling' the benefits of the new approach to patient care to others.

The benefits of this 'selling' style in this study were: the dissemination of the innovation to other wards, units and departments; the creation of a nurse advisory service between the nurses caring for elderly people in the general and psychiatric hospital; the setting up of a self-help education group between the units implementing the change; and the clarification of the nurses' thoughts about the process of nursing and the changes they had achieved (Keyzer, 1985).

Thus, the 'selling' style can be of most benefit when the nurse is dealing with clients who are willing to change, seeking direction, and / or require information to clarify the reason for change.

In the beginning, the change agent may have to provide the direction and information required by the client. As with the 'telling' style, this need for support wanes as the client gains confidence and expertise.

Participating

This style is described in the normative–re-educative approach to change and is the strategy appropriate to the needs of individuals and groups who are motivated, willing, and able to change (*see* Fig. 1.2). Thus a supportive, non-directive style, which permits the participants to control the change and which values their inputs, has the greatest chance of success. Keyzer (1985) further describes such a group in the case study of the implementation of the nursing process in a psychiatric rehabilitation unit. In this case study, the charge nurses provided strong leadership and were supported in the need for change by some, but not all, of the staff. Group norms and values were used by the leaders to initiate support groups for those members of staff who had the ability to change, but were unwilling to do so through a lack of motivation or confidence. The charge nurses, in their roles of change agents, negotiated with the group to make decisions and set goals for the proposed change. In this way new nursing records were created; experimental shift systems were initiated; new attitudes to and behaviour of staff towards the patients were developed. Minimal directives were neither given by the external change energisers (the Nursing Process Development Group) nor were they sought (Keyzer, 1985).

One of the contributing factors to the success achieved by this group was that it had identified the need for change and selected a nursing model and process before the 'telling' and 'selling' strategies of the Nursing Process Development Groups had been initiated. Thus, the 'participating' style is most likely to succeed once the group have identified a need for change and have perceived its relevance to their daily practice (Keyzer, 1985).

Delegating

This style is an extension of 'participating' and is most appropriate for individuals and groups who have achieved a self-directed approach to change (see Fig. 1.2). Indeed, a self-directed, independent learning strategy is a perfect example of the 'delegating' style. It is the one most commonly used for students engaged in research studies. In this strategy, the change agent provides the minimal amount of support and only does so when asked by the group. Normative–re-educative strategies have the greatest degree of success and support the initiatives and independent actions of the individual(s) involved.

Whilst Hersey and Blanchard (1982) and Haffer (1986) perceived these situational leadership styles to be independent strategies, they could be seen to be steps in a continuum. There may be, for example, occasions when the nurse initiates the change by 'telling' the client about it, then proceeds to 'selling' the plan of change, goes on to support the 'participation' of the client in implementing the plan, and ultimately 'delegating' it to the client. Thus, these styles can be part of a problem-solving approach to planned change in nursing practice, education and management. All of these strategies and styles were utilised by Keyzer (1985) in an attempt to assist clinical nurses in implementing the nursing process in a setting caring for older patients (*see* Fig. 1.3).

Summary

The implementation of planned change in nursing organisations is a complex process which can be influenced by the individual's or group's perception of the need for change and its relationship to the daily practice of nursing. Furthermore, nurses need to consider how changes in nursing practice can affect the work of other health care

Group's response to change	Change strategy
Clinical nurses and teachers feel insecure and threatened by change towards implementation of the nursing process.	*Telling* Power–coercive. Statutory Bodies' directives to schools of nursing and midwifery. Policy endorsed by Nursing Policy Group.
Group gains greater confidence but feels insecure because of lack of information.	*Selling* Rational–empirical. Nursing Process Development Group set up to disseminate information and to identify and forge links with pilot areas.
Group gains confidence, but still requires support and information.	*Participating* Rational–empirical and normative–re-educative. Teachers negotiate learning contracts with clinical nurses to support move towards implementation of the nursing process. Groups become involved in study days and seminars on implementing the nursing process.
Motivation grows as group gains confidence in own ability to change.	*Delegating* Normative–re-educative. Pilot areas develop a self-help education programme. Teachers' roles change within the group and assistance is offered only when asked. Group publish accounts of the changes achieved.

Figure 1.3 Examples of change strategies adopted by the author and clinical nurses attempting to implement the nursing process in practice and education. After Keyzer (1985)

groups and how these groups can promote or inhibit the achievement of desired nursing goals.

To ensure the success of any change in nursing practice, education or management, the nurse must negotiate with other health care groups. She or he must be able to convince others of the benefits of change in attaining the goals set out in the organisation's strategic plans. The support for and the collaboration of others is more likely to succeed if the nurse has a framework for practice, which clarifies thoughts on the nature of the change and provides a process to implement the change in a logical and practical manner.

There are three strategies available to the nurse planning change in practice, education and management. These strategies are:

- rational–empirical
- power–coercive
- normative–re-educative.

Each of these strategies may be used on its own, but it is more likely that a combination of all three will be needed to meet the needs of individuals and groups. Furthermore, the focus of the change and the individual's or group's willingness and ability to change may dictate that these strategies be combined with different leadership styles.

These leadership styles are:

- telling the individual(s) to change
- selling the idea of change to individual(s)
- participating in the change process
- delegating the control over all aspects of the change to the individual(s).

Whilst these strategies and styles may be seen as independent approaches to change, a combination thereof leads to a continuum along which the individual(s) may be found at any point in the change process.

The success achieved in implementing planned change will be influenced by the following:

- The active involvement of all levels of nurse and those whose practice overlaps the role of the nurse.
- Open channels of communication which permit the diffusion of the innovation throughout the organisation.
- The involvement of managers in supplying the resources needed to achieve the desired outcomes.
- The involvement of the teaching staff in supportive education programmes throughout and after the period of change.
- The participants' perceptions of the need for change and its relationship to their daily practice of nursing.
- The negotiations of flexible agreements between the change agent and the participants, and between the nursing service and other health care workers whose practice will be affected by the change.
- The active involvement of the participants in all aspects of the process and in setting time frames for the implementation and evaluation of the proposed change.
- The setting of standards and selection of criteria for measuring the outcomes of the change. This includes the individual's or group's evaluation of the success achieved.

Throughout this chapter, reference has been made to three specific nursing texts (Keyzer, 1985; Wright, 1986; Pearson, 1989). These texts have been chosen because they describe and evaluate the conscious application of change theory to the implementation of nursing models and other innovations such as primary nursing in practice and education. Each of these writers selected participating styles (*see* Figs 1.2 and 1.3) to underpin normative–re-educative strategies for change.

In their separate texts Keyzer (1985), Wright (1986) and Pearson (1989) have shown that clinically based nurses can effect change in nursing practice. Each identifies the constraints imposed by low staff:patient ratios, lack of understanding by others of the nature of the change and the distribution of power and control in nursing organisations. These factors do inhibit the progress made, but an understanding of how these variables affect our practice enables us to select different strategies and styles to minimise their influence. In this way, they exemplify that there is nothing so practical as a good theory when it comes to meeting the challenge of change in nursing practice.

References

Bennis, W.G., Benne, K.D., Chin, R. and Corey K.E. 1976 *The planning of change.* Holt Rinehart and Winston, London.

Bernstein, B. 1975 *Class, codes and control, Volume 4, Theoretical studies towards a sociology of language.* Routledge and Kegan Paul, London.

Beyers, M. 1984 Getting on top of organisation change, Part 1 Process and development. *Journal of Nursing Administration* **14** (11), 31. Getting on top of organisation change, Part 2 Trends in nursing service. *Journal of Nursing Administration* **14**(11), 327. Getting on top of organisation change, Part 3 The corporate nurse executive. *Journal of Nursing Administration* **14**(12), 327.

Black, M. 1991 *The growth of the Thameside Nursery Development Unit.* King's Fund, London.

Davies, C. 1980 *Rewriting nursing history.* Croom Helm, London.

General Nursing Council for England and Wales. 1977 *GNC Education policy,* Ref. 77/19/A, HMSO, London.

Haffer, A. 1986 Facilitating change. *Journal of Nursing Administration* **16** (4), 1822.

Hall, D.J. 1977 *Social relations and innovation.* Routledge and Kegan Paul, London.

Hegyvary, S.T. 1982 *The change to primary nursing.* The C.V. Mosby Co., St Louis.

Hersey, P. and Blanchard, K. 1982 *Management of organization behaviour* 4th ed. Prentice Hall, Hemel Hempstead.

Keyzer, D.M. 1985 Learning contracts, the trained nurse and the implementation of the nursing process: comparative case studies in the management of knowledge and change in nursing practice. PhD Thesis, London University.

Pearson, A. 1989 *Nursing at Burford: a story of change.* Scutari, Harrow.

Pembrey, S. 1980 *The ward sister: key to nursing.* Churchill Livingstone, Edinburgh.

Stacey, M., Dearden, R., Pill, R. and Robinson, D. 1970 *Hospitals, children and their families.* Routledge and Kegan Paul, London.

Sugden, J. 1984 The dynamics of change. *Senior Nurse* 1(13), 1215.

Turner-Shaw, J. and Bosanquet, N. 1991 *A way to develop nurses and nursing.* King's Fund, London.

Towell, D. 1975 *Understanding psychiatric nursing.* Royal College of Nursing, London.

Towell, D. and Harries, C. 1979 *Innovation in patient care.* Croom Helm, London.

United Kingdom Central Council 1986 *Project 2000: a new preparation for practice.* UKCC, London.

Vaughan, B. and Cole, A. 1994 *Reflections: 3 years on.* King's Fund, London.

Vinokur, A. 1971 Review and theoretical analysis of the elements of group processes upon individual and group decisions involving risks. *Psychological Bulletin* **76**, 23150.

White, R. (Ed.) 1986 *Political issues in nursing: past, present and future, Volume 1.* John Wiley and Sons, Chichester.

White, R. (Ed.) 1986 *Political issues in nursing: past, present and future, Volume 2.* John Wiley and Sons, Chichester.

Wright, S.G. 1986 *Building and using a model of nursing,* Edward Arnold, London.

2 Theory into practice: some examples of the application of change strategies

Lesley Surman with Stephen Wright

Introduction
Examples of different strategies in the clinical situation
Summary

It has long been an axiom of mine that the little things are infinitely the most important.

Sir Arthur Conan Doyle, *A case of identity*

Introduction

Clinically based nurses can and do effect changes in nursing, constantly and continuously, but frequently without realising or understanding how it happened.

Passing through a hospital, or any centre where caring, management or education is taking place, it is possible to catch snippets of conversation (without intentionally eavesdropping of course!) which make reference to the need, the doing of, or the already having made changes to, existing practices. These come from all levels of staff, in all avenues, that combine to make the organisation which enables the caring of, and the caring for, people to happen. Nurses make up the largest percentage of the workforce among the caring professions. It is therefore important we become aware that we can not only be the subjects of change and innovation, but that we can also generate and perpetuate new ideas ourselves. There is a vast range of constructive ways in which individuals can contribute and participate to produce change and gain the rewards of their achievements.

Mauksch and Miller (1981) identify that 'the status of the individual who suggests new ideas seems to have great bearing on the manner in which new ideas will be accepted'. Sadly this is still true to a great degree. However, changes are afoot, and there are occasions when evidence of this can be seen.

In this chapter, the strategies already identified (rational–empirical, power–coercive and normative–re-educative) will be examined in relation to clinical practice. Short case studies, examples of both success and failure in change, will be given to illuminate the advantages and disadvantages in adopting a particular strategy, either knowingly or innocently. In some instances, a particular strategy adopted has some characteristics of others.

Whilst all case studies are hypothetical and bear no reference to any person or persons known, it is hoped that they present a realistic and recognisable situation. It may be questionable as to whether change is needed, or indeed whether knowledge is advantageous in achieving a smooth, comfortable passage through this delicate operation of achieving change. The answer is undoubtably yes. The past has presented many occasions when the senior management has issued a directive, the junior wanting to be helpful and obliging says, 'yes sir,' then proceeds to moan, be aggravated and even obstructive because they lack the information, knowledge or involvement to make them feel a real part of the suggested change. Instead they become frustrated that they are puppets to be manipulated at will.

CASE STUDY

Harold was a 35-year-old gentleman who was admitted to hospital with a diagnosis of hypertension, obesity and constipation. The treatment he required was relatively straightforward and mainly concerned with education and the introduction of a healthier diet. The difficulties presented required careful re-education and adjustment to his life style. While this may be easy to say, it may be extremely difficult and hard work for any individual to make this adjustment and then maintain it.

On admission Harold was seen by the doctor who told him, 'We will give you some medicine to sort out your constipation and bring your blood pressure down, but you need to lose at least four stone in weight, that means a diet, and you will have to stick to it.' Harold found this rather depressing; he'd been on diets before and had had little success. Now it sounded rather serious. The nurses on the whole were quite nice but they only said the same things as the doctor. Harold began to feel that pressure was being put on him from the people with power. Unfortunately Harold was none the wiser as to how he was going to go about losing this weight; his experience of dieting had led him to believe his life sustenance was to consist of salads! On his third day of admission, Harold found himself talking to a student nurse. This was only her second clinical allocation and she didn't seem bossy or upset with his moans and groans. Harold decided to ask this junior nurse questions to which he had had no answers, and which were now beginning to bother him. The junior nurse didn't have all the answers, but she listened and seemed to empathise with the tremendous upheaval Harold felt was about to change his whole way of living.

Over the following few days the student nurse built up her relationship with Harold and guided by the primary nurse, brought leaflets, cookery books, and ideas to Harold. He began to realise that life was not over. There were foods he could eat, if cooked correctly, his social life wasn't over, he could still go out and have a drink. Taking up exercise didn't mean five laps of the park before going to work, and importantly he didn't have to go it alone; there were groups and clubs which he could join which would enable him to share his agony with others in the same boat.

The student nurse helped Harold adjust and come to terms with the changes he had to make to his life style in order for him to enjoy good health and well-being. She had little knowledge of the strategy of change she was employing, but the inherent qualities and characteristics expected, and quite innocently employed by this nurse, enhanced and nurtured a trusting relationship and promoted self-help in Harold.

This nurse and all nurses have the qualities and abilities to enable them to be change agents. Status on its own should not automatically lead an individual to perceive themselves as a radical/revolutionary change agent. The change suggested may be perceived as small or large, but it should always be given fair consideration and not discredited, ignored or undermined no matter who has offered the idea.

What is important is that nurses are educated and trained in using their inherent talents constructively. They must be given the knowledge to enable them to go forward into the ever changing world of nursing with confidence.

Before change is initiated, the change agent is advised to plan the change realistically, critically analysing the reasons for the change, identifying expected goals and outcomes, and his/her own attitude and that of the target group. Approach is all-important in effecting change. A problem existing for the change agent within nursing is that the target groups focused upon generally cover one, two or three decades of age differences. The training and education of nurses has changed considerably over the years and the acquired perceptions, values, views, opinions and practices of these individuals can conflict with regard to the requirements of each to enable them to accept change or participate in change.

Middleton (1983) identifies that potential nurses are chosen for having 'several basic characteristics which are inherent within a personality; these are in general agreed to be reasonableness, honesty, decency, honour and integrity'. Ethical values and codes of practice espoused in nursing incorporate concepts such as these. We need to ensure for ourselves and our colleagues, that these qualities do not diminish with time.

The behaviour of the change agent is vitally important to the success or failure of an innovation. Change agents who were, and still are, perceived by themselves and respectfully by others as extremely good, innovative, creative and stylish change agents, have been known to attribute to others the resistance encountered towards change, instead of recognising that it is in fact being triggered by themselves. It is a hard and sorry lesson to have to learn through practice, and, in fairness, change agents and clinical leaders are human too! There is a risk that we can fall into the trap of superhood – feeling that we can and should be able to do everything to perfection. It may sometimes be difficult to see and admit that the contributing factor to resistance is produced by oneself, and if this can be achieved, the human support of a peer, colleague and friend can help the pain to dissipate and the 'what to do' to be worked out. The person who acts as a change agent needs to have a high level of self-awareness, not only of how they personally respond, but also how they affect others. The target group need to feel involved and responsible. If the change agent can achieve this, then change will be seen to occur more quickly and smoothly.

The change agent needs to avoid conveying a sense of superiority over others as this inhibits others in the team feeling that genuine participation and empowerment is on offer. He/she may have been the person to identify the change needed, why it is needed, perceive the outcomes of achieving the change, and identify how to do it, but he/she alone does not make change happen. A feeling of trust, corporate effort, shared goals and visions, confidence and competence needs to be nurtured in the group. The change agent must demonstrate an appreciation and understanding of the limitations and capabilities of the individuals who are to change, be involved in, or implement the change. It is therefore very important that the need for change must bear identifiable relevance. The target group must be able to positively identify with the benefits it should promote. They not only need to know why it is being postulated but also the expected goals and outcomes. Unclear change programmes, without understanding the rationale, and with no clarification of actual and possible goals, is one reason for resistance from the target group.

There are, of course, other reasons for the resistance and it is frequently encountered with any movement away from the *status quo*. Insecurity within individuals, fear of the unknown, competition for power or influence, and limited resources may also be contributory factors.

Individuals or groups strive to achieve their personal goals and, therefore, challenge proposed changes. The challenge is not always realistic or justified. It is presented not with the view to how it may help the proposed area concerned, but how it may contribute to the individual attaining their own goals, and thus more influence and power. It is not so long ago that nurses believed once they had completed their training, passed their exams and were admitted to the register, they were then complete products and had no more to learn. Any nurse still believing this is sadly under a misconception and should prepare for an uncomfortable journey through nursing. Recent legislation and policy in relation to nursing has made it mandatory for nurses to accept our responsibilities for continuous updating of our professional knowledge and skills if we are to remain on the register and continue to practise. Each of us has a professional duty and responsibility to keep up to date with the latest findings; research, professional practice and developments. It has become incumbent upon us to keep up to date, not just with the immediate world of our practice, but also with other developments which impact upon nursing practice, such as the enormous expansion in the use and potential of modern telecommunications and computer technology. Not to comply with the computer requirements for practising nurses is not only unfair to his/her colleagues but potentially detrimental to themselves. It has to be remembered, too, that there is an obligation by managers and teachers to enable the nurse to meet these requirements. Ignorance is not accepted as a reasonable excuse, nor indeed is omission of action.

A favoured and much used resistance tactic is based in the past experience reference. If that experience was pleasant, more eagerness will probably be found in attempts to achieve change.

CASE STUDY

It was the custom within this particular unit for the senior sister/ charge nurse to cook breakfast for the staff of his/her ward who were on duty on Christmas Day morning.

The sister on the ward, enjoying this ritual, produced the full cooked English breakfast one year which the staff thoroughly enjoyed.

The next year sister thought they could try something different, a traditional Cheshire breakfast perhaps. The staff would not even contemplate it, 'the breakfast you cooked for us last Christmas was smashing, we'll have the same again this year thanks'.

There was no reason to change, everyone was obviously happy with last year's arrangements, so they enjoyed the same again. If the original experience had been negative, the prevailing attitude towards a fresh approach might have been different.

CASE STUDY

Several years ago, in the formative stages of moving away from the task allocation and towards total nursing care, the 'work books' came under close scrutiny. The outcome was to recommend their removal from practice.

Whilst Nurse Brown, a third year student, was not alone in her disapproval of this change, her past experience produced resistance to the change, and a resulting bad experience.

Since the removal of the 'work book', nurses took to writing copious notes on scraps of paper which they then kept in their pockets for reference. It was the practice of the night nursing officer to do 'a round' with the nurse when she visited the ward at night; name, age, religion, diagnosis of patients all had to be recited. Nurse Brown was so worried about being told off if she did not know all the information that it went down on a piece of paper and into her pocket, to be pulled out when 'the round' came.

Nurse Brown survived 'the round'; tired and relieved she went off duty at 8 a.m. Whilst walking through the hospital, she put her hand in her pocket to get a tissue. On pulling out the tissue she dropped her information-laden piece of paper. Unfortunately, it was found and read by relatives who had been called in to see a patient whose condition had deteriorated and who was referred to on the nurse's notes. The diagnosis of 'Ca Bronchus' was on the piece of paper; neither the relatives or the patient had been told. There resulted much upset and unrest. Nurse Brown was disciplined.

Some years later, Nurse Brown, then qualified, found herself working with a progressive and innovative sister, in an area where the nursing process, primary nursing and other aspects of patient-centred care were well established. Sister James proposed that the care planning system could be advanced by developing a system of patient access. There was no way Nurse Brown could bring herself to work this new practice, her past experience blinded her to any advantages it had, all she felt was acute stress and fear. She obstructed the change in any way she could, overtly and covertly. Eventually she left to move to another area.

The past experience, although not totally related, bore strong enough resemblances for Nurse Brown to view this with only a negative perspective. When faced with a negative response it is helpful to analyse the two situations, identify areas that will be different in approach, execution, and/or expectation, in an attempt to win the unconvinced over before either discarding the idea or proceeding with it.

Achieving change needs careful consideration from the onset; most importantly in the area of communication. Inadequate communication and support from the top level increases apathy and sponsors a lack of involvement amongst the nurses; interest is lost and cooperation diminishes. Whilst there must be agreement on the goals and probable and possible outcome, one must estimate whether this is realistic when considering the requirements to achieve it.

If the time is insufficient, staff turnover is such that it promotes inconsistency and if finances are inadequate to accomplish the change with a degree of success, it is questionable if the change should be embarked upon. Change is threatening to those with the broadest of outlooks, let alone those who cannot see beyond the conclusion of the task in hand. Failure is demoralising and will make attempting innovation and change extremely hard to contemplate within this group again. It is, therefore, best to ensure that, as far as possible, the resources are there to fulfil the change successfully. Starting off with a small scale scheme can be helpful; a quickly achieved goal (and recognition of it) can do much to reinforce the morale of the staff for grander changes to come.

The final form of resistance is passive, which is often inactive and concealed. Inefficient, stubborn or sullen behaviour are all symptoms of passive resistance. It is thought to manifest itself as a result of suffering difficulty in controlling one's own work environment or in directing change for ourselves (Cooper *et al.*, 1987). The change agent, having assessed his/her own attitudes and behaviour and that of the target group, then needs to go on to implement the change, using the most appropriate strategy. As described in the previous chapter, there are choices of strategy to be made.

Examples of different strategies in the clinical situation

Power–coercive (telling)

Change is mostly recognised as 'top-down' directives. We are 'told' what to do, 'when' to do it, and 'where' to do it. Unfortunately the 'why' and 'how' it must be done is often missing. The answers are important though in achieving success in change. Traditional 'top-down' style management appears to be common in the NHS (Price Waterhouse, 1988) which inhibits the opportunity which nurses have to be creative change agents at clinical level.

Many policies, procedures, standards and protocols are still laid down and issued by management in many settings. Staff in the clinical areas are expected to implement them without question, going very much against the grain of the patterns endorsed in this text – of staff empowerment, participation and control. The presentation style of documented procedures has, over the last few years, meant a change. There is a definite, positive and much-needed move away from the directive approach of documentation towards principles as guidelines

CASE STUDY

After publication of the Patient's Charter, a team of community nurses found themselves subject to a series of memos, often quite blunt and directive, from their manager. To ensure that targets were being met, a number of directives were issued to ensure that the nurses timed their visits. There was no discussion with team members, simply a list of requirements about how and when to ensure that patient appointments were kept within a maximum delay of half an hour. The staff felt angry and ignored. The impossibility of achieving this goal with the complexity of their caseloads seemed difficult to convey to the manager whose attitude was very much 'you will do it because it's the rules now, and because I say so'. This was the 'last straw' to many in the team, and the latest in a long line of conflicts between them and their manager. At a group meeting, much anger and hostility boiled over. The manager seemed very much under pressure herself, but refused to give way. The meeting broke up with much frustration and bitterness, and the conflicts continued for several more months, during which several staff resigned to take up jobs elsewhere and the manager eventually moved to another post. The conflicts seemed to have little to do with particular issues, rather than with a particular autocratic style of leadership that left little room for positive relationships and understanding of each other's positions to develop.

While organisational policies and procedures may be set up to protect patients and ensure certain standards, they may be adhered to rigidly or rejected by staff who are not allowed or feel unable to use their initiative, or who resent an 'order' being imposed from elsewhere.

to practice. However, the procedure book 'bibles' exist in many places and nurses at clinical level can find themselves subject to edicts in all manner of ways.

Rational–empirical (selling)

This approach assumes that people are going to view change in a positive manner and work constructively towards it if they are given the basic facts, and so long as there is some evidence that they will derive a degree of benefit from the change. As previously identified, the target groups in the caring field usually comprise members with many differing ages, values, attitudes and experiences. Ways of doing things which are sufficient and acceptable to one individual or group may well not be for others. Using this strategy, the change agent uses persuasion; attempts to sell the proposed change by offering inducements, incentives and rewards, or suggests that new knowledge provides a sound reason for change.

CASE STUDY

Whilst visiting the wards of a rehabilitation unit around the lunch time period, a visiting manager was appalled to see the beds were still in disarray. The ward looked untidy as an outcome of this and the manager was most displeased. Two days later, a memo arrived for the wards of that unit stating that all beds on the wards must be made by 11 a.m.

The staff were upset and angry on receipt of this memo as they had been given no explanation of why this was so essential, and no opportunity to state their reasons for this not being assessed as a priority of morning duties. The memo served only to reinforce amongst the staff that belligerent bureaucracy was still alive and thriving. There was good reasoning for the practice of leaving beds unmade; it was part of the patients' therapy to make their own beds.

The memo was discussed at a staff meeting and the consensus of opinion remained that they would be failing in their responsibility to the patients in maintaining individualised care if they changed their organisation of priorities. Consequently, the majority of beds remained unmade until after 11 a.m. There was no positive outcome from this power–coercive strategy, and no positive change occurred. It did, however, serve to strengthen negative attitudes towards management; trust, morale and the feeling of achievement from work well done were all diminished. Even putting honourable, constructive change proposals to this group of people was met with hesitation, wariness and degrees of resistance for some time after.

The introduction of the nursing process and patient allocation is another example of change which met with animosity (Wright, 1986). Indeed, in some establishments its introduction was of a power–coercive style, which then progressed to the more used rational–empirical strategy to enable any degree of success to be attained. The target group for this change already had many converted members and others who were able to be subagents. It is, however, a good example of how long change can take. The English National Board estimated ten years for the change to be complete, yet there is still a long way to go before it can be said to be established and working to its full potential nationally. There are still individuals who are not convinced of the need for this change, but more have been 'sold' the idea and are enjoying the benefits it brings. Many other instances of change being widely promoted have fallen into this trap, be it nurse practitioner roles or primary nursing, clinical supervision or nursing development units – a great deal of interest is generated for a while, followed by lots of conferences, journal articles, books and courses on the theme, and very soon a bandwagon appears to be rolling. The opportunity for reflection, exploration, education and

CASE STUDY

Following a decision to devolve budgetary control to clinical teams, study afternoons were arranged for ward managers and team leaders to attend where their new budgetary responsibilities and assessment of requirements and expenditure would be explained to them. A lot of time was spent describing the important step and how it would benefit both patients and staff. The incentive was that each ward would receive a percentage of their expenditure savings to be used in whatever way the ward wished. Although this sounded quite attractive, actual figures were lacking (as at the end of the day was the money).

In this instance, not only were the new budget controllers not fully told the whole aim, nor given realistic goals and outcomes, but no one advised them how to go about achieving this without lowering standards. A great moan from many new budgeters was not so much the saving of money, most knew that money could be saved in some areas (although not in the quantities requested nor with the repetition year after year which had been specified), but where the time was to come from? What should they give up in order to meet these new responsibilities?

On the whole, two years later at least, few, if any, ward budget holders are any wiser; they remain bewildered, pressured and disheartened, and very tired. They also remain uncertain as to what their individual budgets were.

This is possibly an instance where little progress was likely to be made, and it is hardly surprising that the proposals were met with a multitude of resistance strategies.

CASE STUDY

Jaqui and her team attended several lectures after the 'named nurse' initiative was announced in the Patient's Charter. It was supposed to be implemented right across the country by 1997, but she was confused about some of the principles and most of the people in her organisation seemed to feel the same way. Everyone seemed to be saying it was a wonderful thing for her patients and for nursing, but was it really going to be that easy? She and her colleague, Gary, felt that they seemed to be well organised along this route already, but how could they be sure? Most of the people speaking or writing about it seemed to be managers or policy-makers, not clinicians like her who would be expected to deliver. Eventually she began to meet up with people who were experiencing similar difficulties, and found that the problems they encountered had been very little aired in the wider nursing media – they decided to write an article for publication to redress the balance. It was not that they were not supportive of the principle, more that they would have preferred a more realistic and honest appraisal of what it was, its problems and benefits so that they could have been better prepared and able to deal with the difficulties when they arose.

gradual adaptation can be lost as we come under increasing pressure to implement something that we feel is being foisted upon us. In the enthusiasm to sell an idea, resistance to change is exacerbated as we begin to feel not so much that something is being sold to us as 'told'. There is a tendency to extol the benefits of the new 'product' in order not to discourage us, but not to admit its limitations or difficulties. Unrealistic expectations can be created followed by disappointment and failure when any proposed change is implemented, only to fall apart when the first obstacles occur for which we are not prepared.

Normative–re-educative

The previous chapter has suggested that this is the most effective strategy in influencing change in the long term. The change agent encourages participation and delegates responsibility. In this strategy, the change agent may be an active or passive member of the group, giving information, advice and direction when it is required and asked for, but allowing the group to motivate and direct itself, with possibly decreasing involvement of the initial change agent as the competence and confidence of the group increases. A classic example of this is described by Manthey (1981) in relation to primary nursing. It did not arise because nurses were told about it and expected to implement it, but because it was a totally new idea and Manthey and her colleagues were to create something new. Essentially, a group of nurses looked at the way they were organising care, and all the problems they were having, and decided that 'there must be a better way'. They arrived at primary nursing from their own experience, intuition and problem-solving, and in doing so created a phenomenon that has spread to nursing across the world (Wright, 1993). The clinical leader – Manthey herself – adopted a style that was supportive and facilitative, as did the local managers, allowing an idea to flourish and grow.

Change always brings new experiences and, as more details are known of how we may go about achieving change, then it is hoped that the experience it gives will be of a positive nature. It is quite exhausting for those with established practices to have to embark on tearing them apart. The approach is all-important in promoting willingness and motivation in members of the target group (the change agents' attitude was discussed earlier). Ownership of the change process generates support and commitment. Success, even in one small arena, nourishes more success, and fosters a 'can do' spirit among the team even when great difficulties and obstacles are encountered. This strategy, it has been suggested, is best used when approaching individuals who are motivated, willing and able to change. Many individuals can, however, be re-educated and re-energised to participate as has been suggested.

CASE STUDY

Bogumila, a nurse working in a hospital in Poland, had been very much cut off from western ideas about nursing. As political changes towards democracy in her country got under way, she was able to access ideas about nursing which had hitherto passed her by. She was inspired by some of the ideas she read about, and she began to discuss them with her colleagues who were willing to try them out, but she also noticed how many ideas in the west were shared by her colleagues and herself. They had already begun making lots of changes because they 'felt right' and not because they had read about or been told about them. They did not use words like 'primary nursing' or 'nursing process', but the principles they had begun following spontaneously were much the same. They set about creating one ward which would pilot some of the ideas they had heard of, and found that they had very much in common with things they wanted to do anyway. Reorganising patient care, to get rid of rigid visiting rules or find a simple care planning method or start setting standards of care, began to flow from this committed team who just wanted to 'do things better'. Fortunately they had a sympathetic matron and hospital director who encouraged them to experiment and innovate, allowing a flowering of ideas and changes to take place in the clinical area.

CASE STUDY

Patrick and his colleagues working in the community were disheartened by so many changes that were happening to their team, and the sense of threat that arose with the reorganisation of the health services with the advent of the trust, the purchaser–provider split and the creation of GP fundholders. How would they survive in this new 'market'? They felt that others had a very limited view of what district nursing involved, and were horrified by the comments from some GPs that they thought it possible to count up how many dressings would need changing, allocate a fixed time for each one, then work out how many nurses it would take to do the job. No-one seemed to understand that district nursing was infinitely more complex than this.

They decided that something would have to be done, and if the market was what mattered, then they would have to be as good as anybody else at marketing what they did. They persuaded their manager to buy in an external nursing consultant to facilitate their work, and in the months that ensued they developed their own marketing strategy to put district nursing 'on the map' and to educate others about what it really entailed. They set up seminars for invited audiences of GPs and Health Authority members, took selected individuals out with them for a day to show them what they really did, provided a resource centre and resource packs with information about district nursing, and set up training days in marketing skills for nurses so that every nurse could turn every encounter, wherever they were, into an awareness-raising session on the reality of district nursing. These and other measures not only helped to transform views about district nursing, but also enthused and energised a team of people who had hitherto felt disempowered and hopeless.

Summary

Whilst being 'told' what to do can be a comfortable way of functioning for many people, the effectiveness of any particular task carried out is of better quality when the individual concerned knows why it should be done in a given way. Effecting change is not so different. As the target groups can be of such diverse characters, the approach, level and strategy adopted must be compatible with their abilities. If resources of any kind are required, the change agent and managers have a responsibility to ensure they are available.

Support is essential, especially in the early stages. Individuals have a vested interest in maintaining the *status quo* in terms of their own ego and power. Change creates uncertainty and anxiety. It questions long-standing and established practices which can undermine the individual's self-esteem. The type of support needed varies for each individual during the course of implementing change. The commitment of the managers and change agents is essential, but support can be gained from the peer group(s) and recipient group(s) as well.

A positive attitude towards achievement of the goal of those involved is essential. Involvement as early as possible is beneficial. In this way, the individuals become interested, their commitment is gained, and the rewards reaped, not just in productivity, but also in the individual's self-esteem.

To return to an earlier example, in many establishments the background work for the introduction of the Named Nurse standard was completed before the target group was approached. Action was often expected without full consultation and involvement of the target group. The instruction to change to what was for some to be a new way of organising nursing was met with much animosity. Involvement of the target group at the planning stage could have alleviated many problems and promoted an earlier attainment of success. The strategy of change adopted in the early stages of any innovation may be different to the style in which it is completed.

The needs and requirements of the target group may change and, with this possible occurrence in mind, change agents should continually be observing, assessing and evaluating their strategy. An innovation such as the Named Nurse, which started with a power–coercive change strategy in many places, has, through time in many establishments, been continued using an rational–empirical strategy. Today, in most instances, the emphasis seems to have shifted to a normative–re-educative approach. Similar parallels can be drawn with many other nursing innovations in the past decade.

That change is inevitable is a fact that we have to accept. The better equipped we are for involvement in its execution, the more likely it is that success rather than failure will be the outcome. This chapter has set out a number of short examples to illustrate some of the principles set out in Chapter 1. It is clear that the change process is far from linear ... often we experience 'three steps forward, two steps back', and the next two chapters will look at some of the rich complexities of managing change and how nurses can work as change agents.

References

Cooper, C., Cooper, R. and Eater, L. 1987 *Living with stress.* Penguin, Harmondsworth.

Harward, D. 1979 *Power: its nature, its use and its limits.* Schenkman, Boston.

Manthey, M. 1981 *Primary nursing.* Blackwell, Oxford.

Mauksch, I.G. and Miller, M.H. 1981 *Implementing change in nursing.* The C.V. Mosby Co., St Louis.

Middleton, D. 1983 *Nursing 1.* Blackwell Scientific Publications, Oxford.

Price Waterhouse 1988 *Recruitment and retention of nurses.* Price Waterhouse, London.

Wright, S.G. 1986 *Building and using a model of nursing.* Edward Arnold, London.

Wright S.G. 1993 *My patient; my nurse – the practice of primary nursing.* Scutari, London.

3 The nurse as a change agent

Stephen Wright

Introduction
Who are the change agents?
The shifting sand effect
Ownership
A 'bottom-up' change strategy

Prometheus by his free will undertook and carried out responsibly his plan, though he knew very well the consequences of his action. He had other alternatives, but he chose the nobler one and committed himself to his decision, which was to help men do better by making them masters of their minds.

Vassiliki Lenara, *Heroism as a nursing value*

Introduction

Why should nurses change (either themselves or the world around them) at all? It seems that the pressures for change are both external and internal. On the one hand, there are the changing needs of society and the political and economic forces which impinge on nursing. Pressure for change may come from governments, or professional organisations. This may be reinforced when those who make use of nursing, the patients or clients, as well as the potential users, find that all is not well with nursing. On the other hand, nurses themselves may come to an awareness that they could not only do things differently, but better.

Not all change is necessarily a change for the better, but we are in a weak position to judge this unless we are aware of who we are and what we do, and are able to articulate it to others. Achieving such a status may take many years, on the long road from novice to expert, as described by Benner (1984), but nurses at least seem to be becoming connoisseurs of nursing, if the explosion of literature about nursing by nurses in the last ten years is anything to go by, as well as the recognition by more and more nurses that it is necessary for us to be able to sell the value of nursing to others.

It is perhaps the failings in nursing practice that give most genuine cause for concern. These might be identified by nurses themselves or those who make use of their services. The opportunity for the latter to express their views should increase with the growing acceptance of quality assurance methods which involve patients and clients. The test of nursing's success therefore seems to come from three directions, as shown in Fig. 3.1.

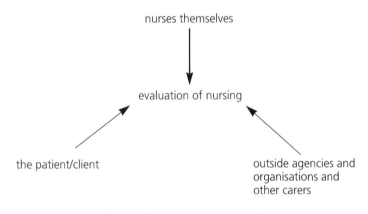

Figure 3.1 Perspectives on nursing

When nurses are required to change their practice, it takes expert nurses to judge whether the change is in the best interests of their patients. Unfortunately, many nurses still lack the knowledge and skills to be able to do this and they find themselves unable to resist negative changes when they are imposed upon them.

The institutional, hospital-based emphasis on nursing this century has produced many deep-seated problems for nursing. Historically, much of the training of nurses has taken place in hospitals (Beyers and Philips, 1971). The dangers of the institutionalised approach to care by the carers, which develops in the 'total institution' (Goffman, 1961), should not be underestimated. Nurses, like any other discipline, can develop an institutionalised attitude to work, just as patients themselves can become institutionalised in the hands of the carers. Once socialised into this attitude, the nurse will act it out. In an effort to bring order and control to the working day, the nurse can inflict upon the patient a degree of order and control which denies the patient even the most basic of human rights, dignities and freedoms.

Martin and Evans (1984) explored many of the failings in such a setting, including:

- negative values related to nursing and patients
- lack of leadership
- lack of development/knowledge of the staff
- lack of resources
- lack of involvement of staff and patients in the decision-making process
- poor facilities, buildings, etc.

Unfortunately, when such problem hospitals have hit the headlines, there has been a tendency to search for scapegoats and to punish the 'evil' staff concerned. However, this may do little to alleviate the problem in the long term unless the nature of the institution is itself challenged. 'Individual psychopathology may have a part, but the issues are both broader and deeper. They are broader in the sense that much turns on the attitudes of society to its weakest members, and the resources assigned to their care; they are deeper in that what may occur is a perversion both of individual motives and of social institutions' (Martin, 1984).

The effects of the institutional approach are not confined to hospitals. Nurses and other carers at work in the community can develop and display similar attitudes as witnessed by the countless media reports into neglect in nursing, residential and social services homes and the patients' own residences. Meanwhile, the regular reports to parliament of the Health Service ombudsman suggest that complaints by patients about impersonal, even inhumane care, are rising. The special hospitals, dealing with the branch of forensic psychiatry, have also been the subject of numerous reports and allegations of ill-treatment in recent years.

Abuse is not always so dramatic or demonstrable, often it is subtle, hidden and carried out in the most well-intentioned manner. The tendency of the nurse or other carer, lacking knowledge, time or resources, is to take control of the patient's life. 'Let me do that for you, it will be quicker' reinforcing dependence, and helping the carer, at least in the short term to 'get through the work' (Clarke, 1978) more quickly.

While the worst excesses of nursing failings (at least those which are reported) are relatively rare, there is no room for complacency. There is a need to be a constant watchdog over the service that is provided, to be aware of what needs changing and how best to go about it, whether it involves us changing ourselves, or confronting the organisation with its own errors and inadequacies.

Who are the change agents?

Change agents may be people who are brought in from an outside organisation to change things, e.g. a consultant from a managerial company brought in to advise on the reorganising of a department. Alternatively, the change agent may be someone who works within the organisation who provides the expertise to make changes. Of course, not everyone wants or is able to change things. Nursing might be seen as being particularly disadvantaged in this theme, not only because we have yet to mature as a profession which can clearly articulate what it is, but also because it is a female-dominated organisation, which has not traditionally been taught the skills of leadership. 'It is all very well being urged to provide leadership, but difficult in practice, especially as so few of us have been adequately prepared for such a role. Nursing particularly suffers from the fact that qualities such as leadership are not seen as socially or culturally appropriate for the women who comprise over 90% of its workforce' (Salvage, 1988; Rafferty, 1993).

What does seem clear is that the potential to be a change agent lies, to a greater extent, in every nurse. Each nurse may approach change in a different way and with varying degrees of enthusiasm.

Rogers (1962) (Fig. 3.2) suggests that any given body of workers will vary in their responses to the challenge or threat of change. The leaders in change and innovation come from a small minority, with their followers gradually adopting the new ideas over time until only a few change resistant workers or 'laggards' remain.

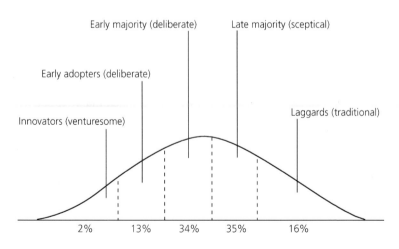

Figure 3.2 Change – the responses by the staff (total number of staff in the work setting on a scale of 0–100%). After Rogers (1962)

The change resisters can produce disharmony in the setting, hold up progress, or form 'cliques' to support one another. What is taking place in the change setting, as it takes on new values and new directions, may leave the resisters feeling isolated. Ultimately, if the change becomes adopted permanently, they may vote with their feet by leaving. Thus, in some settings where change is taking place, the organisation has to be prepared that some staff may leave when they finally feel they cannot be a part of the team.

However, it is important to avoid seeing Rogers' model too simplistically. It can be argued that there are no laggards or venturesome 'types', rather these are just forms of behaviour that we can expect from people at any one time. They are not constants and it would be inappropriate to label anyone under any of these categories as being a particular type of person. Someone may behave in a laggard way at work, but be completely different in another setting. Likewise, I may normally be quite venturesome when it comes to change in practice, but if I have left home that day having had an argument with my partner, received some bad news in the post, crashed the car and lost my wallet, then maybe I will not feel too venturesome that day! The behaviours are therefore not stable, but subject to all kinds of situational variations.

It also has to be remembered that the above scale is heavily value laden, i.e. the innovators are 'good' the laggards are 'bad'. However, not all change is for the better, so, depending on our point of view, resisting some changes might be considered good. It can also be argued that resisting change performs a useful function too, for we are all then tested and learn from it, and those who would pursue change are more likely to be required to be certain of their case, produce the evidence for change and reflect upon the correctness of their course.

Perhaps what needs to be recognised is that everyone has a part to play, it being too idealistic to assume that everyone will be an enthusiastic supporter of change. Often the question is asked by those involved in introducing change – 'What do I do with those who will not come with me?' It seems that there are a number of options to consider. First of all Rogers' model gives us some clues about how people can be expected to respond to proposals for change, and in so doing suggests that we can use different approaches with different people. The people who respond with early adopter behaviour will need little from the innovator, except information and support, as they will quickly participate. Those who fall into the early majority category might need a little more time to listen and learn, but will follow on because they 'respect' and support the innovator and will follow their suggestions because they tend to trust him or her. Those who are more sceptical may need to see that the innovation actually works – a visit to another site where it is in operation, a copy of the research evidence and so on. The resistance to change that takes the form of laggard behaviour may manifest itself in anything from mild obstruction or unwillingness to participate to outright hostility and/or subversion. They may protest, form pressure groups or attack the changes, especially in the absence of the principal innovator. It is this last group where the greatest resistance can often be felt, which needs to be overcome by allowing more time to adapt and for education or finding specific ways in which they can have a particular role to play. However, it may be that as suggested above, they may ultimately leave or even various disciplinary methods may have to be used. The author has experience of working in a very institutionalised setting where it seemed that at one time the great majority of the staff behaved in laggard ways. Gradually over many months more and more staff began to commit themselves to the change process, but a small number had to be brought into line using power–coercive methods, and in the end several were dismissed. Anyone who has experienced such action will tell of the painful and difficult process that this involves. This illuminates, as suggested in the first chapter, that the most successful change agents are able to use a variety of strategies to effect change rather than adhering obsessively to one particular strategy. However, it needs to be remembered that instances which reach the point of discipline and dismissal tend to be very much in the minority, and that those who behave in laggard ways perform a service too, and not just in forcing reflection and reappraisal of what is to be changed. The innovators' skills, knowledge and compassion for others are also brought into the equation. It is relatively easy to work with those who are 'on our side', much more difficult with those who appear not to be, and yet who teaches us more about ourselves and demands the best use of our knowledge and skills? In addition, for change to succeed, not all nurses need to be 'on board' to the same degree, but looking at the nursing development unit movement as an example it seems that once a setting has about 60% of the staff 'moving' (Lewin, 1958) then resistance is largely overcome.

Rogers' model can help us to look at the change setting and ask how might different staff be expected to respond, so that we can plan different approaches in advance. It also helps us to make decisions about what tactics to employ with different people as the behaviours arise. Of course you might start by asking yourself how you think you might respond to the idea of change and see where you fit on Rogers' continuum at the moment! Furthermore, the innovator is not always in a position of power, so how can we change things when we are feeling innovative, and yet we are blocked by a more senior member of staff? The power–coercive approach is not an option, but other methods of persuasion through reasoned argument and evidence (selling) or helping to bring people together to start the changes (normative–re-educative) are available to us. Forming a 'conspiracy' will be discussed a little more in the next chapter. Sometimes it is not possible to start change because we simply do not have the knowledge, power or influence with those who have power over us. Long-term 'Machiavellian' strategies may be deployed, or we may chose to go and work elsewhere. If the latter is not an option, then perhaps all we can do is continue to take care of ourselves and our patients to the best of our ability, cherish what we do well, and continue to find ways to make changes and develop ourselves until the time is right.

There is an obligation on the part of the change agents and those who support them to involve the whole team in the change process wherever possible, regardless of the chosen strategy, and endeavour to bring even the most resistant along with them through education, support, rewards, and so on. Ultimately, however, some will go, but this should not be a major problem as those who replace them, if aware of the setting to which they are going, are likely to already accept the values of the organisation in which they have chosen to work.

The words 'change agent' have been used frequently so far, and it is appropriate to look at this concept a little more. We tend to use the notion of 'change agent' in relation to the ones who are actually leading the changes – the innovators or venturesome ones. Ottaway (1980) analysed the different types of change agents and develops Rogers' (1962) ideas further. In effect, everyone is a change agent in some way, but participating in different ways. Again the reader might ask 'what sort of change agent am I?' when reading the next sections.

Change generators

1 Prototypic, the 'hero' type, changing hearts and minds with passion, enthusiasm and charisma.

2 Demonstrative, of which there are three 'subspecies':
   (a) 'barricade' demonstrators, the demonstrators at barricades or on the streets, often at the front line of conflict;
   (b) 'patron' demonstrators, benefactors of the change process, e.g. giving money or appearing at meetings to offer support;
   (c) 'defender' demonstrators, representatives of those who will benefit from the change, e.g. an elderly person speaking up at a public meeting to support changes in a local hospital.

Change implementors

Once a need for change is recognised they are brought in to implement it. They may be:

1 External change implementors such as nurse consultants invited in, e.g. on a 'freelance' basis to help the staff.

2 External/internal change implementors, e.g. a nurse teacher working on one site, but visiting others to assist with developing new ideas.

3 Internal change implementors work with their own peers and colleagues within the organisation to change things, e.g. a practice development nurse in a trust.

Change adopters

These fall into three types:

1 The prototypic change adopter – their task is to be the first adopters of the change in the organisation.

2 Organisation maintenance change adopters – they can be very resistant, but may adopt the change in order to preserve as much of the rest of the system as possible.

3 Product (service) users change adopters – the change in the service is adopted by the user, e.g. the patient.

Ottoway's interesting taxonomy indicates that the change generators are often mistrusted in the organisation, that they like to effect change quickly and move on, and that they have very well thought out values. For simplicity, the words 'change agent' are used in this text to refer to change generators unless otherwise stated. Change implementors work on the 'felt need theory', i.e. helping people to change because they have come to feel that they want to. They are often seen as more trustworthy, working with colleagues to sell their ideas.

The change adopters form the mass of change agents. Their task in the process is to take up the change, but they are often unaware of their role in the process. This reaches down through all grades of staff and ultimately to the patient or client. When this succeeds, patient and staff satisfaction are in harmony; when it fails, there can be problems.

CASE STUDY

The staff on a ward gradually adopt a progressive approach to care, removing restraints on elderly patients. The patient's relatives complain that the staff 'don't care' any more because they do not appear concerned with safety. The change, the need for it, or the philosophy behind it, has not been explained to the relatives and the patient. Two differing world views are in conflict because there has been no dialogue between the two parties to achieve shared understanding around a proposed change.

Rogers' and Ottoway's models may seem rather complex, but they do offer an opportunity for the nurse who would be a change agent to assess:

- where do I fit in among these types? Am I a particular one, or do I have qualities akin to many? If so, how will my colleagues perceive and react to me?
- where do all my colleagues fit into these models? Who will support and who resist? What strategies can I use to deal with these?

The shifting sand effect

Imposing change in any setting can be likened to taking a walk along a beach when the tide has just retreated. The wet sand is inviting, ripe for having new impressions made upon it. Thus some nurses try to change things. Entering upon virgin territory, they stamp their mark upon the staff and the way they work. The footprints are deep and obvious, like those on the wet sand. But, as the innovator walks on, the footprints gradually fill in, the sand returns to what it was before, and nothing has changed. Imposing change in any setting may be success-ful in the short term but, ultimately, it fails.

Scheff (1967) described the concept of 'front line organisations' – the ability of groups of workers to ignore or manipulate the orders that the boss has given. Thus, the innovator may believe that change has occurred because they ordered it but the reality is that, in their absence (when they leave, or simply go 'off duty'), the system reverts to what it was before. How many clinical leaders have implemented a change on a ward or unit and gone off for the weekend suspecting that, as soon as their backs are turned, the staff are 'up to their old tricks again'?

Ownership

If the 'shifting sand effect' is to be avoided, then real change must be owned by those who use it. Ownership of the change process and its results must be the prerogative of those who are doing the work. By owning the change, the staff come to feel it is their decision. It is their property. We tend to cherish, care for, and preserve those things which we ourselves have created.

The new norms and values which come to pass in the situation where change has occurred are far more likely to remain permanent if the staff themselves feel they have created them. Such a process requires a skilful change agent who helps them to produce change from the 'bottom-up', thereby avoiding the pitfalls of 'top-down' charge.

A 'bottom-up' change strategy

As has been suggested, it is possible to bring about change in people's behaviour by a direct authoritarian 'power–coercive' approach, i.e. by telling them how to do things differently. However, there are risks in this model. When the authority moves on, or becomes less effective, then there is a danger that a reversion to old norms and values takes place. Change can only become permanent if the desired values and practices have become a permanent part of the people in the care setting. An institutional framework can be broken down, but an alternative resilient framework must take its place if the changes are not to be swept away when the innovating change agent departs. For alternative goals and values to be reached for people to come to a different view of their world a more egalitarian strategy is a necessary tool. Lewin's (1958) classic change theory defines 'no change' as a 'quasi-stationary equilibrium . . . a state comparable to that of a river which flows with a given velocity in a given direction during a certain time interval'. He describes social changes as comparable to a change in the velocity and the direction of that river, and sees the change process as having three basic steps:

- *Unfreezing* when the motivation to create some sort of change occurs, the impetus for this coming from three possible mechanisms:

1 *Lack of confirmation or disconfirmation*, i.e. the awareness of a need for change because expectations have not been met.

2 *Inducing of guilt or anxiety*, i.e. uncomfortable feelings because of some action or lack of action.

3 *Psychological safety* when a former obstacle to change has been removed.

- *Moving* when change is planned and initiated where cognitive re-definition occurs to look at the problem from a new perspective either through 'identification' or 'scanning' (the former solution provided by a knowledgeable peer: the latter solution found in a variety of sources).
- *Refreezing* when change is integrated into the value system and stabilised into a new equilibrium.

In order to 'unfreeze' existing norms and 'move' the staff to 'refreeze' into new norms, a tool to do the job is required. Many alternatives are available, and producing change in nursing is often a designated role for many practitioners, managers and educators. The idea of embodying change strategies in a specifically designated person, the change agent, to produce change is accepted by many authors on the subject (Lewin, 1958 and Rogers, 1969 among them).

Ottaway (1976, 1980) identifies a change strategy using a change agent, with the ability to use Lewin's model, who can work to implement change from the 'bottom-up'. He further identifies a strategy where managers and educators act in support roles to the on-site change agent, who, in this instance, works with staff and patients over a period of time (it may take many years!) to produce change (Fig. 3.3) (see for example Pearson, 1989; Black, 1991; Turner-Shaw and Bosanquet, 1991).

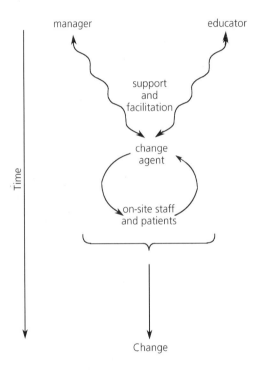

Figure 3.3   'Bottom-up' change strategy

Clearly, if any one element in this model is lacking, then the chances of success are hindered if not blocked completely, e.g. the manager is unsupported.

Ottaway (1976) identifies six crucial factors for this type of change:

- *Bottom-up*: there is participation of the 'shopfloor' workers and the change may move up into the rest of the organisation rather than the reverse.

- *Pilot site*: the new norms are practiced here first rather than across the whole organisation at once. A site is chosen where the staff are willing to participate.
- *Training follows change*: participator begins to feel need for new knowledge and skill which is then supplied rather than trying to change people for new skills and expecting them to apply them.
- *Contracting*: the staff decide on the how, what, and when of the change for their own small unit.
- *Made to order*: the change process is fitted to the unique individual setting and not applied as a preplanned package everywhere.
- *Felt need*: the change is determined by the needs the staff feel, rather than imposed by outsiders.

These key elements are incorporated into various steps of the change process.

Step 1: Agreeing goals – a vision for the future

The staff get together and agree new goals and directions, however large or small they may be. The staff participate in developing and sharing a vision for the future embodying their views on how their work could be better. What are we trying to do? How can we improve things? The skills of the change agent are seen as instrumental in guiding the ideas and generating questions, without seeming to impose plans. The person may, for example, be a ward sister, but the important features are that they have knowledge and skill, work on-site with the staff, and are seen to be part of the team without necessarily directing it.

Step 2: Make a diagnosis

How is the work organised? What is wrong? What are the aims of the organisation or unit? What are each staff member's abilities? What resources are available? What is the management style like? In other words, the change agent assesses the nature of the organisation in order to make a plan of action.

Step 3: The design of intervention

This should be done by the people who have to make it work and they should map out what will be changed, how it will be done, and even for how long.

CASE STUDY

A nurse on a unit wishes to implement primary nursing in her setting. At a staff meeting she mentions the subject (Who is interested? Who isn't?) and gets the staff thinking about it. Some agree it is a goal they would like to learn more about. A few more meetings take place (often at the pub or someone's home as it can be difficult to confer a meeting at work!) including meetings with the night staff (Step 1).

The aims and the problems are discussed. Currently, care seems a little impersonal, sometimes less organised. The theory of primary nursing looks like it might help solve these (Step 2).

Plans are drawn up for allocating patients, agreeing case loads, who will be a primary nurse, who an associate. The organisation of the ward is reviewed, and an experimental implementation period of six months agreed (Step 3).

A date is decided to begin primary nursing. Weekly meetings are held to review difficulties, as well as informal discussion sessions at each shift change, as need arises. Problems are reviewed, case loads adjusted, grievances aired (Step 4).

The staff find they need to know more. Lectures on accountability, visits to other units, meetings with other primary nurses are requested. More books and literature are obtained (Step 5).

Things seem to be progressing. The staff say they enjoy the new sense of responsibility and sister is more free to support the staff. Patients like having 'my nurse', and say so. The manager notices the happy atmosphere on the ward and compliments the staff. Relatives praise it. Complimentary letters are received (Step 6).

Some staff move to other areas to pass on their ideas. Other staff come to the unit to seek advice and return to their own areas to try it out themselves (Step 7).

For simplicity, each of the steps has been reduced, but, as may be seen, they are highly complex acts, fraught with difficulties. The change process is rarely so linear and logical, and this theory will be explored in more detail in the following chapters.

Step 4: Implement the intervention

Put the plans into action, and have review sessions as matters progress.

Step 5: Skill training

Enable the staff to learn the new skills which they begin to feel they need, e.g. better communication skills, more knowledge on a nursing problem, how to use a computer, etc.

Step 6: Reinforce new norms

Talk about success and congratulate each other! Give praise when it is due and be wary of criticism. Rewards might be offered, e.g. study leave, bursaries, etc.

Step 7: Replicating

Transferring the experience and knowledge and repeating the steps on other sites.

In effect, the application of Ottaway's strategy is a call to 'proletarianise' the process of change in nursing. The avoidance of this 'top-down' authoritarian approach encompasses the transfer of the governance of change into the hands of those whose lives are most affected by it. The 'pedagogic dialogue' (Freire, 1973) which takes place between change agent and the on-site staff is seen as crucial in generating ideas and changing old norms into new ones. The staff are helped to become aware of their situation and guided in the transition to alternative methods. In so doing, they own their change process and, therefore, have an investment in its success and retention.

References

Benner, P. 1984 *From novice to expert.* Addison Wesley, California.

Beyers, M. and Phillips, C. 1971 *Nursing management for patient care.* Little, Brown, Boston.

Black M. 1991 *The growth of the Tameside Nursing Development Unit.* King's Fund, London.

Clarke, M. 1978 Getting through the work. In: Dingwall, R. and McIntosh, J. (Eds), *Readings in the sociology of nursing.* Churchill Livingstone, Edinburgh.

Freire, P. 1973 *Pedagogy of the oppressed.* Writers and Readers Publishing Cooperative, London.

Goffman, I. 1961 *Asylums.* Penguin, Harmondsworth.

Lenara, V. 1984 *Heroism as a nursing value.* Sisterhood Evniki, Athens.

Lewin, K. 1958 The group reason and social change. In: Maccoby, E. (Ed), *Readings in social psychology.* Holt, Rinehart and Winston, London.

Martin, J. 1984 *Hospitals in trouble.* Blackwell, Oxford.

Ottaway, R.N. 1976 A change strategy to implement new norms, new style and new environments in the work organisation. *Personnel Review* **5**(1), 1315.

Ottaway, R.N. 1980 *Defining the change agent.* Unpublished research paper. University of Manchester Institute of Technology, Department of Management Sciences, Manchester.

Pearson A. 1989 *Nursing at Burford; a story of change.* Scutari, Harrow.

Rafferty A.M. 1993 *Leading questions.* King's Fund, London.

Rogers, C. 1969 *Freedom to learn.* Merrill, Columbus, Ohio.

Rogers, E.M. 1962 *Diffusion of innovations.* Free Press, New York.

Salvage, J. 1988 'Facilitating model based nursing'. Unpublished paper given at Gateshead School of Nursing Models Conference.

Scheff, T. 1967 *Mental illness and social processes.* Harper and Row, London.

Turner-Shaw, J. and Bosanquet, N. 1991 *A way to develop nurses and nursing.* King's Fund, London.

4 The change obstacle course: additional perspectives on the change process

Stephen Wright

Introduction
The culture of change
Forming a conspiracy
Resistance
Clinical leadership
Planned change: additional dimensions

It is often safer to be in chains, than to be free.

Franz Kafka, *Metamorphosis*

Introduction

Kafka's phrase is a salutary reminder to nurses of the dangers of change both to themselves as individuals and as a group. As the previous chapter has suggested, not everyone approaches change with the same degree of energy and commitment. Using the problem-solving framework can help in organising change, but rarely does it work so neatly or in such a linear fashion. Nurses and the world they work in are far too contingent. The work of change is always messy and unpredictable to some degree. Effective change agents understand and accept this principle, for those who seek a perfect, simple and linear path in change are more likely to exhaust themselves in pursuing an impossibly perfect and illusory path.

Many nurses in many settings have tried to change what goes on around them, only to find their energy dissipated and their enthusiasm burnt out when confronted with the killing tripartite; obstructive management, unsupportive educators and resistant colleagues. Under these circumstances, it is little wonder that many keen and committed nurses have given up in despair and resentment. They discover that 'when you stop banging your head against a brick wall, the headache goes away'.

Change is difficult, if not impossible as many nurses have found to their cost, when they have decided to 'go it alone', or have been thrust in by the management of the institution to an undesirable setting to sort things out. Georgiades and Phillimore (1975) illustrated how the 'hero innovator' is not as effective a change agent as is often assumed. When used by the organisation to put things to rights they may exhaust themselves, may move on leaving things to revert to the *status quo*, or they may fail and become discredited. In the process, they discredit the change process and reinforce the view that it is impossible to change the situation anyway.

The culture of change

Toffler (1973) writes of the 'death of permanence'. We live in a society where everything is open to question and threatened by change and, moreover, where such change is accelerating. The health care system cannot remain isolated from this, nor can its nurses. The health services themselves must now accept a new culture (the *status quo* is not an option), and this requires that change, the acceptance of it and the practice of it, must be part of the normal day-to-day activities of the organisation. The acceptance of this new culture has not occurred wholesale or simultaneously in the various levels of the health services. There is a risk to nurses, as individuals or in small groups, who seek to change things in their setting when other parts of the organisation are stuck in the preservation of the existing order mould. Changing practice at clinical level has difficulty in expanding and progressing if the total organisation has not accepted the culture of change. It does not render change impossible, but it does produce limitations. The change agent must be aware of these factors in order to limit the obstruction they can present, limit the damage that can be done, and how to overcome or get around them.

Praill and Baldwin (1988) note that 'Rather than the continuation of frenetic, isolated and disjointed clinical practice and innovation attempts, a system is required which is itself innovative. Responsibility for innovation should be corporate, rather than invested in key individuals'. They suggest, like Toffler (1973), that change itself needs to be an inherent part of the total system on which nurses work.

Furthermore, nurses must not expect that they or other professions can be the sole determinants of change. Many innovations blowing through the health services are led not by those who work in them, but are a product of rising demands and expectations of the users of the health services – patients, clients, residents and so on. Indeed, this is seen as preferable; 'A structure is required to facilitate the development of active consumer-led systems, which demand change for the benefit of client groups' (Praill and Baldwin, 1988). Increasing attention has been paid in recent years to notions of empowering those who use health services through, for example, giving access to medical records, issuing statistical data on the performance of Trusts, setting up advocacy and inspection schemes and so on. Indeed, the notion of patients as consumers with certain rights, with health care staff working in partnership with them, was embodied in the issuing of 'Patient's Charters' from 1992 onwards in the UK. If partnership with and empowerment of patients have become concerns of the day, then where do nurses fit into this scheme of things? They are providers of care (and therefore must respond to consumer-led demand). Yet, in some respects, they are also consumers either as potential patients themselves, or of the workplace which provides them with a living, as well as (hopefully) job satisfaction. Thus some organisations, such as the National Association for Staff Support, have advocated the setting up of staff charters as well as to set out the rights and responsibilites of those who work in the health care system (NASS, 1993).

If the recent trend towards primary nursing in the UK is taken as an example (Audit Commission, 1992; Wright, 1993), whence comes the push for change? There seems to be a double-edged blade at work, but which came first, or whether both arrived in tandem, it is difficult to discern:

• Patients as consumers demand more personal care, more information, more accountability from care providers.
• Nurses' professional aspirations, dissatisfaction with less personal modes of care, more control over individual patient care.

Perhaps the culture of change in health care is at its most potent and most successful when the needs of both provider and recipient have shared aspirations. There seems little doubt that such innovation is most successfully accomplished in a climate which encourages it, that is, when the system in which nurses work has accepted that change is an inevitable and desirable part of its culture. Creating settings where 'change is a way of life' (Salvage and Wright, 1995) is one of the principal goals of Nursing Development Units (NDUs), and for this reason a later chapter has been devoted to them (Chapter 5). A setting seems to become ripe for change when a number of factors seem to come together as previous chapters have indicated – such as the presence of an innovator, new demands on the service, a sense of shared vision and purpose among the staff for a better future and so on. The organisation as a whole benefits from this climate for change and the 'ripeness'. It seems, for example, that the desire to remain 'in chains' is a response to the threat of change and all the upset it can bring. Studies have shown, however, (Orton, 1981; McClure *et al.*, 1983; Price Waterhouse, 1988, Black, 1991) that working climates where staff feel they are supported, where they feel they are learning, and where they feel they can innovate, are more likely not only to recruit nurses, but to retain them as well. 'Indeed, what does come through rather vividly from the data is that magnet hospitals have the total picture in place: the management is supportive of professional nursing practice within the context of a teaching/learning environment' (McClure *et al.*, 1983).

It appears that the ideal climate for nurses, those they serve, the organisation in which they work, and those who manage it, is achieved in a setting where innovation is the norm. Nurses in such a setting are not necessarily seeking and using power for power's sake, rather they feel that they are not powerless. Being involved, feeling listened to, knowing that management is responsive and not oppressive, appear to be important feelings to nurses which support them in their work and make them feel free of their chains to innovate.

However, it may be wondered how many nurses today work in a climate such as this. Perhaps not the majority, many might answer, although Toffler (1973) appears to offer some hope in his model. The 'accelerative thrust' of change will eventually overwhelm all institutions which fail to respond to the needs of their workers and their consumers. Like the incidence of Canute against the waves, the tide cannot be held back. Sadly, because change in some areas lags behind that in others, some nurses might have to wait a little longer and struggle a little harder for their professional aspirations to be realised.

Forming a conspiracy

If the nurse as a change agent cannot change things alone, then he or she must enter a conspiracy. This involves working together, networking and generating support among like-minded colleagues – nurses and other members of the multidisciplinary team, service users and other carers – to create a context where the pressure for change builds up until it becomes an unstoppable force. The word 'conspire' has its origins in the Latin (*con*: together; *spirare*: to breathe). To conspire requires groups of nurses and others to come together in a shared understanding and common purpose. In so doing, they have more strength to overcome obstacles, they can share and develop new knowledge, and can draw support from each other. Using the models of Rogers and Ottoway cited in the previous chapter, an example would be of the change generator and change adopter on one unit reinforcing one another to overcome the influence of laggard behaviour.

Introducing new norms into a setting is about getting everyone to take on board these values. In some instances, division of the opposition may accelerate the process! However, working together towards shared goals is both rewarding and more likely to produce success as the rabbits in *Watership down* (Adams, 1972), or the comrades of *The hobbit* (Tolkien, 1966) discovered. The notion of groups working together, tapping each other's strengths and supporting each other's weaknesses is a classic model whether it be found in the Bible among the disciples or the revolutionaries in Marxist theory. Working together, having a role to play and drawing the best from each other, seem successful elements of any change strategy.

Resistance

Conspiracy may help to overcome the resistance to change, but a more potent weapon is knowledge. Resistance initially has its roots in fear – fear of doing things differently, of losing privileges, of feeling inadequate or ignorant. Managers can feel threatened, for example, when staff undertake things they do not know about, while others can resist new practices because they do not understand them.

Giving staff the knowledge of who they are, what goals they are aiming for, and how they can achieve them, is an important part of the process. Some of these aspects are dealt with in the case studies (Chapter 6) for example, emphasising the need to 'get people together' so that ideas, knowledge, fears and hopes can be shared. This incorporates a wide-ranging programme of staff development, teaching and promoting self-awareness. It includes the use of many educational strategies; from providing library facilities, courses and conferences, to workshops on communication skills. Pearson (1989), for example, has explored the use of drama in attitude changes in the Oxford Nursing Development Units, along with a variety of other strategies. Purdy *et al.* (1988) detail a similar process in the Tameside Nursing Development Unit. In this way old norms can be 'unfrozen' when new knowledge challenges the established way of doing things, and staff can be helped to 'move' into the new way of being, by development strategies which assist 'refreezing' into new norms. Open dialogue and knowledge exchange may also reduce resistance, reassuring staff that the planned change will not bring redeployment or redundancies, for example, or, if this is likely, providing information about staff protection.

Any nurse who has tried to innovate will probably have encountered many of the classic comments offered to resist change:

- We've been doing it like that for years!
- I'm too old to change!
- The patients wouldn't like it!
- We've done it before and it didn't work! We haven't got the money / staff / time!
- It's not that simple!
- But we work in the real world!

CASE STUDY

'We got together (myself and the two enrolled nurses) to see what we could do about the blockages to change. There were three staff in particular who seemed to have dug their heels in. Every time they got together on duty things seemed to get more difficult. They seemed to undermine what we wanted to do. I don't mind admitting that we plotted. The simple logic of managing the off duty so that they never got together worked wonderfully.' (Ward Sister.)

'I was very much on my own at work, everyone seemed to want to stay with tried and tested methods, which basically meant keeping the patients locked up as much as possible and keeping them well controlled with drugs. I found a lifeline in joining up with colleagues working in the same professional group as me in the RCN – just getting together, feeling I was supported, bouncing ideas around and helping me with evidence and ideas to help move things forward at work. I felt I was not alone, that there were other like minded nurses who could help and guide me.' (Charge Nurse in a mental health unit.)

Exasperation when encountering such remarks is common and, in retrospect, may be humorous. However, they are signs of the very real fears that colleagues can have about change. These fears can only be overcome through:

- Education, providing staff with the knowledge and skills they need to do things differently.
- Time, letting people 'unfreeze, move and refreeze' at their own pace (*see* Chapter 3).
- Reinforcement, using praise when it's due when success, however minor, is achieved.
- Appropriate methods, different people will respond to different approaches to change (*see* Chapter 3). Select the approach according to the behaviour being demonstrated.

Resistance, however, may take more sinister forms than mumbled procrastination. It may, in extremes, move into open hostility, resentment and anger. It may produce conflicts with colleagues other than nurses (witness, for example, the reaction of some medical staff when nurses have refused to help with ECT (electroconvulsive therapy)). In addition, it may put the person pushing for change in conflict with the organisation in which he/she works, e.g. the effects on the 'whistle blowers' in institutions (Martin, 1984), or with their professional bodies and staff organisations. One well known example in the early 1990s was that of Graham Pink in Stockport, who became a *cause célèbre* when he protested about staffing shortages in his hospital. He came into conflict with his employer when he went to the press and subsequently lost his job. While he achieved a degree of fame as a result, and the difficulties of the whistleblower were highlighted, much controversy surrounded the accuracy of his claims, and not all his colleagues supported him. The impact on the care of the patients appears to have been minimal. What this case and others like it teach us is that the 'lone voice' is subject to considerable stress and threat, can be ignored or suppressed, and is of doubtful effectiveness in achieving change. A far more effective approach seems to be to engage colleagues and organisations in the process, although it may well be that whistleblowing is the only option in some circumstances and needs to be balanced against the risks it entails. Anyone entering the process of change needs to have a clear understanding of their professional boundaries and accountability. Nurses continue to be frequently involved in whistleblowing incidents, perhaps because they are faced so directly with the consequences of inadequate care. Perhaps such a strategy is best seen as a last resort when all other channels for change have been explored and failed. The risks to the individual under such extreme circumstances cannot be overemphasised, and although such incidents appear to be relatively rare, they need to be balanced with the possible effectiveness in terms of bringing about desired change at mimimal cost.

CASE STUDY

The boss looked horrified when I mentioned that I was thinking of letting the patients have access to the nursing notes. I spent quite a few weeks giving him information, talking it through, so that he fully understood the reasoning behind it and the prospects. I didn't make a move in that direction until I felt sure he understood it all and would support me.

(Charge Nurse in a community unit.)

For most nurses day-to-day change at clinical level rarely comes into the category of some of those which hit the headlines. It is more likely to be characterised by the daily frustrations of petty obstacles and gnawing frustrations. Planned change is therefore essential to minimise the conflicts which can occur (*see* Chapter 5).

Clinical leadership

In the past decade, a proliferation of media comment has documented an apparent malaise in nursing leadership. A general view is espoused that nursing lacks leaders who inspire the great majority of nurses, offer a clear vision for nursing or are effective in securing the voice of nursing in the circles of power. Nursing, it is alleged, has yet to break away from the medical hegemony and, as a discipline whose workforce is dominated by women, now finds its already disadvantaged position being squeezed on a new front – the rise of new model management in the health services.

There seems to be added confusion in nursing itself – uncertainty of who leaders are, what leadership is and what is their purpose (Rafferty, 1991). A variety of efforts in the late 1980s and early 1990s sought to remedy this perceived problem – mostly by providing specific leadership development to selected nurses. These included, for example:

1 The 'fast-tracking' programme of the former Mersey Regional Health Authority.

2 The 'Leaders Empower Staff' course developed between the Institute of Nursing at Leeds and an independent company headed by Marie Manthey (Creative Nursing Management), well-known for her work in the field of Primary Nursing.

3 The Department of Health sponsored programmes in MBA studies.

4 The RCN's collaborative programme with the Institute of Nursing in Oxford, now based at the RCN's Institute of Advanced Nursing Education in London.

5 A recently developed programme at the King's Fund Centre in London, sponsored by Johnson and Johnson.

These are a few examples of the type of programmes on offer, aimed quite specifically at developing leadership skills in a profession perceived to be lacking them. The pressure to accelerate these developments seems, in part, to have come from the increased sense of threat to nursing in times of great change, not least the reorganised NHS, the increasing emphasis on 'cost-effectiveness' and the questioning of nursing roles, and a growing sense of powerlessness among nurses in decisions which seem to directly affect themselves and their patients – be it re-grading exercises, skill mix reviews or the development of support worker roles. In a climate where events seemed to be increasingly beyond the control of nurses, where what power nursing had (already less than other groups in health services) seemed to be slipping away – the calls for clear leadership seemed to increase in direct proportion to the perceived decline of nursing's influence.

Yet, as Rafferty's (1991) research has indicated, there is no clear consensus in nursing about what leadership is or who the leaders are. There does seem to be a recognition that existing management courses have not been the answer and that leadership in nursing raises very different issues and dimensions of knowledge and skills.

In times of uncertainty, when there is a widespread belief that changes are afoot, where there is a sense of being in little control, then there is a tendency to search for solutions – often those which are quick fixes and easy to understand. The rush toward leadership development in nursing may have been subject to such influences. 'Nursing has problems – where are the leaders to sort them out?'!! This perhaps simplistic approach, although understandable as a knee-jerk reaction, may produce added difficulties:

1 It allows the great mass of nurses to 'opt out' of the problem-solving, i.e. the problems are so great we need leaders to sort them out, so that means I personally don't have to do anything – they're the leaders' problems not mine.

2 Selection of people for leadership programmes may be on the basis of dubious criteria, perhaps because a potential leader has been 'talent spotted' by the hierarchy and encouraged to participate in a course. This runs the risk of leadership programmes being seen as something for an elite group. It may also reinforce the myth that leaders are born (born leaders therefore get spotted and encouraged early on) and not made. This may be OK for the 'born leader' but allows everyone else, yet again, to abrogate the part they themselves can play, i.e. 'It's OK for her, but I'm not a born leader so there's no point in me learning'. There is no evidence that leadership qualities are inherited or belong to one particular type of person.

3 Perspectives on leadership have come almost exclusively from sociological studies and commentary from industrial and political arenas. Very little in-depth study has been applied to nursing. The industrial/political models may not be the most appropriate for nursing, not least because they tend to look from the hierarchical perspective of the great leaders being in (or on their way to) top

positions. If nursing is unique, as is often claimed, and if its subculture is different from that of, say, medicine or management, do we need to develop alternative models for nursing which arise from its peculiar and particular context, influences and nuances? Should nursing necessarily develop leaders and leadership programmes which arise from the reflection in the essentially narcissistic mirror offered by modern (masculine) managerial models?

Much of the drive to foster leadership in nursing has focused on producing nurses destined 'for the top' – the leaders for the professional groups, civil service departments and executive boards of tomorrow. The great mass of nurses, while influenced by (in a myriad of ways) and looking to such leaders, will inevitably remain largely remote from them. And yet it could be argued that there is a need to pay attention to leadership at clinical level, where enormous numbers of nurses, working in teams, might benefit from enhanced leadership. Indeed, little distinction seems to have been drawn between wider organisation leadership roles, and leadership of groups of nurses (and patients) at the service delivery end of the spectrum. All nurses may be in positions where they take the lead in some way – whether it be the community nurse who manages the care of his/her case load and the colleagues who work in a support capacity, or a midwife leading a team of colleagues or facilitating ante-natal classes, or a nurse in a ward who is a ward manager, team leader in primary nursing, or supporting a patients' self-help group. Leadership skills spill over into all manner of nursing roles, yet they are often invisible and assumed to be achievable without specific preparation. Alternatively, it is assumed that such knowledge and skills can be adequately obtained in standard 'line management' courses. The decline in availability of the latter may be symptomatic not only of change in NHS educational opportunities, but also their lack of effectiveness in meeting the real needs of nurses at clinical level.

At the same time, nurses have increasingly adopted the title 'clinical leader' (Vaughan and Cole, 1994), stimulated not least by the King's Fund Nursing Development programme. The acknowledged effectiveness of clinical teams led by a clinical expert seems to belie Handy's (1994) definition of the average British team – that is, a team of people frantically rowing backwards being told what to do by the only person who does not know how to row! Clinical teams deliver patient care, and, despite the many fears and fractures of current services, seem remarkably effective – perhaps in spite of rather than because of the system in which they work in some instances.

Many of the following leadership traits could be ascribed to any leadership position, but there are some which appear unique to clinical nursing, and others where the difference is not so much one of whether they are present or absent, but of the degree of emphasis needed for clinical leadership:

- The leader as visionary – has a strong sense of and commitment to the nursing setting. Is adventurous and works to create the context for the vision and nursing ideals to emerge. Is a 'frontier' person, pushing back the boundaries of nursing practice and exploring new territory. Plans ahead and is able to 'read the runes', translating the vision through action into reality. Works to make it happen at all levels.
- The leader as vision sharer – inspires and awakens others to share the vision, to explore their own visions, and to work towards them. Is able to articulate the vision through clear written and verbal communication. Also recognises the limits of this sharing, that the leader's vision can never be completely taken on board by others. The leader's vision and some facets of it may remain shrouded to others simply because it is the unique creation of the leader in their own head.
- The leader as servant – works to help others develop and put into practice their own vision and ideals, builds relationships, facilitates the growth of others. Knows when to lead from the front, but also when to fall back and let others take the lead, enabling and empowering them to do so. Accepts others as they are, yet works to help them on their own path of development. Respects others and accepts the moral imperative, as a leader invested with many powers, to use that strength to care for and nourish others. Builds and supports the team and its individual members. Like a flock of geese in flight, the 'V' shape is not coincidental – the lead goose creates air turbulence which makes the flight path of those behind easier. When the leader tires, or another wishes to take the lead, he or she can fall back with grace to let others lead for a while.
- The leader as clinical expert – is a nursing 'savant' – marrying art and science, reason and intuition in expert practice in nursing. Is able to set an example of clinical excellence, a 'connoisseur' (Benner, 1984) of nursing and the health system. 'Knows what they are talking about' and is able to demonstrate best practice to others. Is a clinician first and foremost and not a desk-bound nurse. Also 'knows what they do not know' – recognising the limits to their knowledge and practice.
- The leader as change agent – a teacher, listener and risk taker, the leader is an expert in the management of change. Uses their situation, knowledge and skills to help make nursing better. Has the survival skills to help them through the quagmire of change.
- The leader as diplomat – knows 'the system', what makes it tick and how to find a way around things to get the best for patients, staff

and to pursue the vision. Has political 'nous' – knows who the stakeholders and power holders are. Able to get things done, knows when to press on and when to back off. Understands the checks and balances, the power relationships and 'art of the possible'. Is politically as well as clinically 'savant'.

- The leader as inspiration – has drive, energy and motivation, and combines all the leadership qualities to inspire and energise others. Transforms the work settings and the relationships therein from an 'it' (Buber, 1937) (an impersonal place, indifferent, no sense of commitment) to a 'thou' place (a place of sharing, investment, participation, personal investment) where people enjoy being and working and with which they identify. The leader exhibits trust, authority, honesty and constancy and engenders hope, to build a setting where people can feel involved and secure. Clinically and in their leadership qualities, the leader becomes a role model to others.

- The leader as a centred human being – is comfortable with themselves, their strengths and limits. Has a belief in, understanding and awareness of the self. Takes care of the self (*see* Chapter 7) to maintain physical and psychological stamina, and has moved beyond playing the 'victim' or 'martyr' (giving themselves constantly to nursing until there is nothing left) (Snow and Willard, 1989). In knowing their limits, the leader is not an island, but seeks to give help when it is needed, networks with peers for support and is not afraid to reach out to others for guidance ensuring, for example, that they gain clinical supervision for themselves as well as providing it to others. The leader's values are well clarified (about nursing, the self, others, other aspects of life). He or she has little time for 'presentism': 'I have to be at work all the time doing everything, it cannot function without me', but is able to let go, stand back, delegate and take care of the self and other aspects of their time. In being centred, the leader is available to others, yet does not fall into the hero or martyr drama. Knows that they are constantly changing and growing themselves. Draws on values, including spiritual values, that provide a deep well of strength and support. They inform, guide and energise the centre, so that the leader does not exhaust him/herself by constantly giving of the self with no inner resources to call upon. The leader is in harmony with the self, balancing masculine and feminine values and qualities. In being in balance/centred in themselves, the leader recognises that this puts them in the best position to help others. The leader in right relationship with themselves is best placed to help create right relationships in the wider world. Such a person becomes a light which draws others to them, but the leader is aware that sometimes this can repel as well. Some fear the light illuminating, as it may, their own weakness, shortcomings or wounds.

- The leader as 'head and heart' – the centred leader recognises that being in harmony within themselves is essential to creating harmony outside. They are able to guide with qualities of justice, fairness and compassion which inform their normal decision-making and which inspire respect and acceptance from colleagues. The leader has immense power (in themselves and invested in them by the organisation) and this may be abused if it is not grounded in moral action.
- The leader as ordinary – is not projecting themselves as a highly charged charismatic super-nurse, the leader displays qualities which draw others to them, engage their support and command their respect. They know when to laugh and cry, show humility and vulnerability, make mistakes, share concerns and difficulties. By being human and showing their humanity, while still being the leader, they encourage others to be themselves, to become centred, and then develop their own leadership qualities.
- The leader as manager – sees management skills as adjuncts to leadership and not their arbiter. The leader is more than a delegatory organiser, project manager, skill developer and so on. The well documented skills of negotiating, problem-solving, teaching, researching and so on are only part of the story. The leader recognises that these management skills are just manifestations of the inner qualities of the leader. The skills come from the person, and it is the personal qualities that this chapter has focused upon.

Leaders lead change, that is one of their primary functions, and clinical leaders with the qualities listed above, are a potent source of effective change at clinical level. Any person possessing all the above qualities might indeed be deemed 'superhuman' – they are a taxing and demanding schema. Leadership is not just about roles, but inner qualities. Many people occupy leadership roles at clinical level, yet fail to lead, at best only managing. The leader needs all of the above qualities to be effective as a change agent, but does not have to be a perfect human being. Indeed some of the qualities of the leader are the arts of 'knowing what I don't know', 'being comfortable with myself', or recognising that 'I am always changing and growing'. Thus the effective leader does not necessarily require *all* these qualities (for then, they would indeed have some claim to being 'superhuman'!), rather they are in the business of becoming them. The qualities are incremental – the more each person possesses, the more advanced their leadership technique becomes. A steady accumulation of qualities as we refine them along our own journey of personal and professional growth is the foundation of the effective clinical leader. We cannot be a leader by accident, we must choose it – and that choice comes with a lifelong commitment to personal and professional growth which may enhance the whole of our being – physical, mental, emotional and spiritual. While we may act as change agents and clinical leaders, the roles are not just about being effective in the world, but also about our own personal growth, development and fulfilment.

Planned change: additional dimensions

The change process, as described in the previous chapter, is a fairly linear and logical series of steps. This provides us with a framework for planning and implementing change, but it cannot cover all eventualities. In reality, the 'human element' can defy the most rational of processes, adding new complexities and uncertainties. Turrill (1988) identifies seven factors which change agents must consider:

- *Agreeing the core purposes of the organisation.* Setting the philosophy or statement of mission which makes explicit 'why we are all here' and 'what we want to achieve' – the vision for a better future.
- *Sharing a vision of a better future.* Enough colleagues have to share the same vision of the aims of the change which may be years ahead.
- *Operating principles.* Setting out the values, what is important and what is not, to help guide the nurse when faced with uncertainties.
- *Mapping the environment.* Identifying the implications for change on other groups and working out where resistance might come from.
- *Transition management.* Working out how you will manage the journey from where you are to where you want to be in the change process.
- *Resistance reduction.* Working with power groupings/individuals maintaining communication.
- *Seeking commitment.* Winning people over, identifying key groups and individuals.

Many avenues are open to us which can bring people together and stimulate involvement in the process of change and in decision-making. Setting standards of care using groups of professionals can stimulate innovations in practice, as can working in quality circles, various professional forums and policy-making groups. Shared governance and patient-focused schemes, which seek to devolve decision-making to those at clinical level and challenge existing professional and organisational boundaries can generate changes. So too can simply getting together with colleagues, either informally in a social setting or more formally at a team meeting, which stimulates challenge, reflection and dialogue. Methods such as these have many things in common which support successful change:

1 People are brought together to look at what they do and to question it.

2 The sense of threat is minimised as people feel that the challenges come from within the group and are not being imposed from above.

3 The group can determine its own pace and method of change.

4 Coming together in dialogue, often with the presence of a facilitator, helps to pool and generate ideas, and build trusting relationships.

CASE STUDY

In our unit we believe that every patient has the right of choice in his/her care.	= Agreeing the core purpose of the organisation.
We want to provide choices at mealtimes, move away from rigid routines, give access to nursing and medical notes.	= Sharing a vision of a better future.
No patient will have any treatment or care without first being given the opportunity for informed consent.	= Operating principles.
Consider the implications of the code of conduct, maintaining confidentiality, possible conflicts with management, doctors.	= Mapping the environment.
Set up a working group to study the opportunities. One person to research and document progress. Develop new nursing notes.	= Transition management.
Meet with managers, doctors, colleagues. Discuss with relatives and patients. Provide written information.	= Resistance reduction.
Offer staff development programme, teaching, study days, improve job satisfaction.	= Seeking commitment.

This chapter has explored a number of additional themes in relation to the change process. While various models and strategies may offer us a logical framework for action, the reality of change, as has been suggested, is rarely so smooth and linear. Any nurse setting out on the path of change is taking a journey into the unknown to some extent. The ideas discussed so far have sought to provide a map to help with the route; but help is all they can do. That is what can make change so exciting and stimulating. When all the factors have been thought through, planned and practised, in the end there is still an element of adventure, of exploration. In using the logical process of change, it is also necessary to accept the element of the intuitive. The former is the scientific component, the latter the artistic. In the change process, both are necessary parts!

While the 'hero innovator' is a questionable myth, what cannot be overestimated is the real courage needed by *all* nurses who undertake change. In that sense, all nurses who act as change agents are heroes or heroines. Heroism is not just found in the grand acts of history, it is also found in every nurse who attempts to overcome difficulties, however small. As Lenara (1981) notes: 'The goal of the hero and the goal of the nurse coincide. The goal of the hero is to transcend what threatens. And the goal of the nurse is to transcend the obstacles which emerge, from outside and within herself, to threaten her nursing ideal'. This notion of overcoming inner and outer obstacles, of personal development as well as effecting change in the wider world underpins the work of the change agent and clinical leader, some of which will be illustrated in the case studies in Chapter 6.

References

Adams, R. 1972 *Watership down.* Puffin, London.

Audit Commission. 1992 *The virtue of patients.* Audit Commission, London.

Benner, P. 1984 *From novice to expert.* Addison Wesley, New York.

Black, M. 1991 *The story of the Tameside Nursing Development Unit.* King's Fund, London.

Buber, M. 1937 *I and thou.* Clark, London.

Georgiades, N.J. and Phillimore, L. 1975 The myth of the hero innovator. In: Kiernan, C.C. and Woodford, F.P. (Eds), *Behaviour modification with the severely retarded.* Associated Scientific Publications, London.

Handy, C. 1994 *The empty raincoat.* Arrow, Sydney.

Lenara, V. 1981 *Heroism as a nursing value.* Sisterhood Evniki, Athens.

Martin, J.P. 1984 *Hospitals in trouble.* Blackwell, Oxford.

McClure, M.L., Poulin, M.A., Sovie, M.D. and Wandelt, M.A. 1983

Magnet hospitals: attraction and retention of professional nurses. American Academy of Nursing, Kansas City.

National Association for Staff Support 1993 *Staff Charter.* NASS, London.

Orton, H. 1981 *The ward learning climate and student nurse response.* Royal College of Nursing, London.

Pearson, A. 1989 *Burford; a story of change.* Scutari, Harrow.

Praill, T. and Baldwin, S. 1988 Beyond hero innovation: real change in unreal systems. *Behavioural Psychotherapy* **16**, 114.

Price Waterhouse 1988 *Nurse recruitment and retention.* Price Waterhouse, London.

Purdy, E., Wright, S.G. and Johnson M.L. 1988 Change for the better. *Nursing Times* **84**(38), 345.

Rafferty, A.M. 1991 *Leading questions.* King's Fund Centre, London.

Salvage, J. and Wright, S.G. 1995 *Nursing development units.* Scutari, Harrow.

Snow, C. and Willard, P. 1989 *I'm dying to take care of you.* Professional Counsellor Book, Redmond, WA.

Toffler, A. 1973 *Future shock.* Pan Books, London.

Tolkien, J.R.R. 1966 *The hobbit.* Unwin Books, London.

Turrill, T. 1988 *Change and innovation. A challenge for the NHS.* Management Series 10. Institute of Health Services Management, London.

Vaughan, B. and Cole, A. 1994 *Reflections: 3 years on.* King's Fund Centre, London.

Wright, S.G. 1993 *The named nurse, midwife and health visitor.* NHSE, Leeds.

5 Nursing Development Units

Stephen Wright

Introduction
Setting up an NDU – minimising the pain of the process
What is an NDU?
Summary
Appendices

It's the possibility of having a dream come true that makes life interesting.

Paulo Coelho, *The alchemist*

Introduction

Nursing Development Units (NDUs) have been mentioned in previous chapters and considerable interest has arisen in recent years over the arrival of NDUs on the British nursing scene. Are they just a new nursing fad that will disappear in time? This chapter will look at some of the defining factors and then place them in any strategy for change.

The history of nursing is littered with fashions – ideas that were going to help solve all our problems. NDUs are in danger of being seen in that light. They are not panaceas but one way to help bring improvements and innovation in nursing. They are one piece in the jigsaw puzzle of an overall strategy for developing nursing. We have already discussed such strategies in this book, and here the NDU model is discussed because it has become so popular in recent years.

Two centres indicate their origin in the UK. Oxford saw the development of the Burford and Beeson Ward Units in the early 1980s. At about the same time near Manchester, the Tameside NDU was set up and continues to function in the Care of the Elderly Unit eventually becoming the largest NDU. Support from the King's Fund Centre has produced a gathering momentum in the creation of NDUs – with funds made available from the Sainsbury Trust – four more were created in 1989. Thirty more, with funding (£3.2 million) from the Department of Health, were also set up under the aegis of the King's Fund Nursing Developments Programme during 1991/1992. This programme has now been completed and a substantial body of research has emerged about the effects of NDUs (Black, 1991; Turner-Shaw and Bosanquet, 1991; Cole and Vaughan, 1994; Christian and Redfern, 1996).

With this support, notably an injection of funds, NDUs were created more rapidly and with less difficulty than in those areas where they have had to grow more slowly and with no additional funds (as in the Tameside example).

The Oxford and Tameside experience has now been well documented (Wright, 1987a,b; Pearson, 1988, 1992; Purdy *et al.*, 1988; Pearson *et al.*, 1992) and it is perhaps not insignificant that the two persons originally appointed to head up these units both pursued the same Master's programme at Manchester University Department of Nursing. It seems that the knowledge base for change is as important as the change itself. Recent research into the four King's Fund/Sainsbury Trust supported NDUs and the Tameside NDU (Turner-Shaw and Bosanquet, 1991; Black, 1993) have illuminated the nature and value of these changes in improving the quality of patient care and staff motivation, morale and skills.

A significant and earlier text produced on the issue (Pearson, 1983) provides a sound basis for initial thinking about NDUs and these ideas were developed further in more writings (Salvage, 1988; Wright, 1988, 1989, 1992; Barber *et al.*, 1989; Punton, 1989; Black, 1992; Vaughan, 1992; Salvage and Wright, 1995).

There are many ways to change nursing practice, and NDUs are but one option. For example, standard setting and evaluation, creating a change agent, project work or educational programmes can be used as alternatives. However, the NDU model suggests that by focusing directly on and innovating in the practice base of nursing, long-term meaningful change in nursing can be achieved.

Setting up an NDU is itself a complex process; and a few essential steps need to be considered.

Setting up an NDU – minimising the pain of the process

1 Build knowledge on the subject among your colleagues and yourself first. Attend workshops on the subject, read the relevant literature, visit an NDU, seek advice from people experienced in the

field, e.g. clinical leaders in NDUs, or King's Fund Network. Lobby. Discuss. Debate.

2 Spend time sharing ideas at team meetings, and building up a concensus of what an NDU is. Ask yourselves, and answer, the following questions:
   - What is an NDU – are we clear about it?
   - Why do we want it?
   - How will it help us?
   - What will it do to improve patient care/outcomes?
   - What alternatives for innovation can we use and would any of these be better to achieve our goals than an NDU?
   - Who will be the clinical leader?
   - What do we expect the NDU to do? (Identify at least ten things.)

3 If you're sure an NDU is the right way forward for you then set up a small coordination team to produce an action plan. If not an NDU, in what other ways can you develop practice?

4 Once an action plan has been agreed, produce clear written proposals about the NDU – what it will be/do; results expected; projects planned; education links; evaluation plans, etc.

5 Keep the dialogue going with team members, educators and managers so that everyone is up-to-date on the direction.

6 Agree proposals with the team/the organisation.

7 Create an advisory board to guide (but not manage) the NDU. Involve especially clinicians and others whose support is needed – doctors, chief executives, etc. Let someone who also supports the NDU and who has influence within the organisation chair this committee.

8 Allow time for all this process to be pursued – perhaps 12–18 months.

9 Consider applying for grants, special funds, etc., if this is necessary to boost resources for research and projects, for example.

10 Clarify and review the philosophy, objectives/goals of the NDU. Set up a work plan detailing objectives, completion dates, strategies, lead persons and so on. Review this at every coordination meeting of the team.

11 Consider including a team-building strategy before and after the NDU is under way.

12 Make sure everyone who wishes has a role to play – make the contribution explicit in your work plan. Try to ensure that everyone is 'included'.

There are many ways to develop nursing, and NDUs are but one of them. The task is to identify an appropriate setting and goals, but if an NDU is not the right way forward, then other means of developing nursing – such as practice development teams, staff development programmes, clinical projects and so on should be set up.

What is an NDU?

A Nursing Development Unit is a centre for creative nursing, where change is planned and accepted as a way of life, where nursing practices are soundly based but open constantly to challenge and review. It experiments in nursing and explores its boundaries, expanding the knowledge and practice of nursing. It acts as a clinical laboratory where the boundaries of nursing can be explored, yet is a 'safe haven' for innovation in practice, where the risks involved in change can be controlled and managed. It adopts a philosophy which believes that nurses, patients and other carers can unite in partnership to promote high quality nursing care and that nursing can be a healing, therapeutic act in its own right.

To achieve its goals, an NDU is clinically based where nurses are with patients or clients, other carers and other team members. Indeed, the work of an NDU is driven by the clinical staff. The development and educational process, equally available to all, is a 'bottom-up' phenomenon and coordinated by the presence of a specific clinical nurse leader. The NDU is not a response to a 'top-down' approach from managers and educators.

The NDU has the specific goal of producing high quality patient-centred, professional nursing practice, working effectively and efficiently with other members of the multidisciplinary team. The primary goal is double-edged, for it is in tandem with the commitment to develop nurses. An NDU therefore acts to promote these aims simultaneously.

How does it differ, for example, from the 'good' ward or team of nurses, midwives or health visitors who are trying to innovate to improve patient care?

Defining the NDU is not without controversy. The Nursing Developments Programme at the King's Fund Centre developed a 'recognition' scheme (King's Fund 1994). Some settings, such as the Institute of Nursing at Leeds, have set up accreditation schemes. It has been argued (Mangan, 1992) that unless some form of accreditation is introduced, then the concept may be exploited by the unscrupulous or may be diluted when there is no clear consensus as to the nature of NDUs. When the King's Fund NDU programme was under way, several hundred applications for funding were received. Funds for only

30 were available. This led some to feel, falsely, that they had been rejected and were not NDUs, rather than the fact that they did not fit certain specific criteria to obtain funding.

The movement is a growing one. If the numbers of units which have given themselves this label, plus those in the King's Fund network, are added together the total seems to be over 300 by 1996. This does not take account of many units which seem to be NDUs by any other name, but for various reasons have chosen not to apply the title. It is very difficult to apply strict criteria to define this growing body of NDUs. Indeed, too rigid an approach may seek to confine or restrict what is, in many respects, a nebulous concept. One of the advantages of loose boundaries to the NDU concept is the opportunity for flexibility and to develop variations on a theme. No two NDUs are exactly the same and using defining factors may be inappropriate to different countries and different cultures. For example, one factor recently cited as a defining principle is that the NDU has direct links with a higher education setting. In some countries, such opportunities for nurses simply do not exist.

However, given these factors, is it possible to describe the principles which underpin the 'theme' of the NDU? Some aspects may be very difficult to define. There may be a risk of producing reductionist check lists which, with seeming objectivity, enable us to say 'yes, you are an NDU' or 'no you're not'. NDUs are driven by clinical nurses who are often passionately involved in the living world of nursing practice. Measuring such passion and involvement objectively, and the climate it produces, can be extremely problematic. Thus, the following suggestions for judging what is or is not an NDU are extremely tentative. They are based on the experience of many nurses involved in the NDU movement, but they are not exhaustive. Some may be considered more important than others – for example, the absence of a clinical leader may rule out a setting being defined as an NDU. On the other hand, having a nurse in a defined role as clinical leader is not a guarantee that that person is able to foster the culture of the NDU. Furthermore, in some settings, the clinical leader may be the budget holder for the nursing workforce and the available development monies. Is being a budget holder an essential prerequisite, or can an aim to achieve this be acceptable within the defining factors of the NDU? Alternatively, are there other approaches available? Some factors seem to fall in the 'must' category, while others may be interpreted more flexibly, and some suggestions as to their priority are indicated in the following list.

In addition, it needs to be remembered that using an accreditation framework may stimulate change itself (e.g. nurses realise that one factor needs working on that they had previously overlooked). 'Who' accredits needs to be considered. Do nurses simply judge themselves against documented criteria? Is peer group review possible? Can external assessors from authoritative bodies be used? How long should the interval be, before re-accreditation is necessary? Can acknowledged experts in the field be brought in to conduct a review? Each of these approaches has advantages and disadvantages and a combination of approaches using both internal and external validation seems the best way. However, in the final analysis, no one has copyright or monopoly of the title 'Nursing Development Unit'. Any group of nurses can, in theory, set themselves up as an NDU. However, if they do, there clearly are consequences to be faced as the work they do will ultimately be put to the test, be judged by their outcomes, or challenged by others, if not themselves.

With the above points in mind, it seems that the following criteria can be used to help determine whether a setting is an NDU or not.

1. Nursing as a therapy

Nurses in an NDU recognise the value of nursing as a therapy in its own right (MacMahon and Pearson, 1991). By combining instrumental with expressive skills (Benner, 1984), nurses strive to demonstrate that they not only 'care for' people, but also 'care about' them (Dalley, 1988). Thus, it is not only what nurses do with patients, but how they do it which contributes to healing and well-being. In so doing, nurses contribute to patient care by not only helping them to 'get better' but also to 'feel better' (even while dying) (Kitson, 1988). The symbiotic nature of these concepts is recognised, e.g. patients may receive various treatments to help them get better, but the outcomes are improved (i.e. fewer complications, complaints, etc.) where patients also are helped to feel better. Some NDUs may have 'nursing beds' – beds managed by nurses where patients are admitted and discharged where the primary therapy that is needed is nursing. In the NDU the value and primacy of nursing practice are fundamental to all its work.

2. Nursing and NDU autonomy

The work of the NDU is based on the above approach, as it seeks to explore nursing's therapeutic boundaries. Areas of nursing practice which are autonomous are recognised and developed. The NDU itself is autonomous in its work in the setting in which it exists. Similarly, the NDU develops nursing roles which promote autonomy for individual nurses.

3. The NDU is clinically based and owned and led by clinical nurses

The NDU may be part of any health care organisation and is specifically and explicitly committed to the development of nurses and nursing. It may be based in any speciality, in hospital or community, in the public or in the private sector. The NDU focuses on a specific area of nursing practice and is governed by nurses in practice. Its philosophy, ideas and innovations are created and driven principally by the nursing team. Managers and educators have a supportive and facilitative role in the NDU, but they cannot create one or control it by 'top-down' instruction.

4. Size

The size of the NDU may vary, but usually it is located in a specific speciality and focused on a small unit or team. All of the early King's Fund supported NDUs have followed this theme, usually being based on one particular ward, for example. However, it may eventually expand as nearby settings affiliate to its work and philosophy. The early Tameside NDU began on one ward in 1981. By 1986, nine wards and a day hospital were including themselves under the umbrella of the NDU. The liaison and expansion is planned and agreed by all the nursing teams involved.

5. Planning the changes

The innovations in the NDU, and the development of the NDU itself, are not haphazard. An explicit strategy of change is planned and pursued (Wright, 1989). Individual responsibilities within the team for the change are clarified. The objectives of the NDU are agreed and explicit, and a timescale included. The changed plan emphasises a 'bottom-up' approach – involvement of and control by the clinical nursing team, rather than 'top-down' management control. Change in the NDU is a way of life. The NDU becomes a clinical laboratory, constantly open to new ideas and practices, testing and researching them. It is not a static entity but continues to evolve. The main elements of the change strategy include those endorsed in this text, such as:

6. The nursing culture

The NDU places strong emphasis on the development of a team spirit. There is a general sense of 'we are all in this together' and a focus on open communications with each other, participation in decision-making and democratic management styles. The shared philosophy, goals and values become the foundations of the team in the NDU. The shared commitment to change is the driving force of the NDU. It is this culture – the spirit of innovation, passion and excitement about nursing and its possibilities – which is one of the cardinal features of the NDU.

7. A nursing philosophy

The NDU team collectively define and document their philosophy of nursing. From time to time they revisit and review it. The philosophy embodies the team's values about nursing, their goals and aspirations. It forms a basis for a shared vision for nursing and helps to bring a

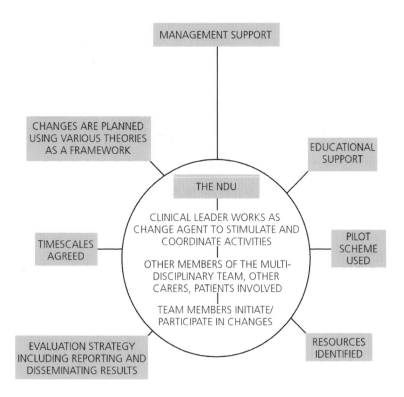

Figure 5.1   The NDU – main elements of the change strategy

cohesive and coherent approach as the NDU pursues its goals (see example in Appendix 5.1).

8. A nursing model

The NDU itself may be seen as a model of nursing in action. In defining its philosophy, actions and focus, the NDU team begin to define a model of practice relevant to their speciality. The NDU may use a formal established nursing model in its work (e.g. Orem, Rogers or Roper, Logan and Tierney, etc.), or it may adapt them. Alternatively it may set about building and defining its own nursing model. Whichever the case, the NDU is able to be explicit about the nature of the model which guides its practice, and recognises that, like its philosophy, this will evolve over time (see Appendix 5.2 for example).

9. Exploring nursing boundaries – innovation and researching

The NDU becomes a clinical laboratory, where nurses explore the nature of nursing and its practice. This may cross a wide range of possibilities from formal longer term research, supervised, for example, by a university nursing department to small scale projects to complement a new practice. All are nursing-led. A continuous stream of activity is planned in the NDU programme. Often, many projects may be under way simultaneously. As one finishes, another begins. All the staff are involved either taking the lead on some projects, participating in others or simply 'getting on with the work' to free time up for others to give attention to their projects. The number, breadth and scope of the projects under way is one of the cardinal features of the NDU. Other settings may pursue one or two innovations and/or studies; the NDU undertakes many continuously. All the projects are characterised by a planned approach, incorporating realistic timescales, identifying resources and the roles each member of the team plays. Nurses in NDUs explore practice by applying nursing theory. At the same time, they develop nursing theory from their practice experience. Traditionally, in nursing it has often been assumed that theory can be taught to nurses who then apply it to practice – NDUs are an example of the principle that innovation in practice can generate new theory.

10. New roles

As the NDU explores practice, it expands the body of specialist knowledge. It may also create new nursing roles to meet newly identified therapeutic needs or to help improve the focus and quality of existing nursing approaches.

11. Application of research

The NDU not only conducts its own research projects, it seeks to apply the results. It also has a strategy to ensure that there is research awareness among the team. Research findings that are relevant and applicable to the setting can themselves be identified and applied. For example, some members of staff may attend courses and conferences on research, others agree to produce reviews and précis of research for the team, a journals club may be formed – and so on.

12. Clinical leadership

Every NDU has an identified clinical leader. This person is an experienced and expert practitioner who motivates, guides and coaches team members and the NDU along its course, usually acting as the principal change agent. The clinical leader is directly involved with the nursing team and in nursing practice. He or she would, preferably, also have control over the NDU's budget resource and staffing, including staff performance, appointment of new staff, etc. Alternatively, there must be agreed protocols with an appropriate manager to ensure that decisions about these features are carried through collectively and cooperatively. Developing the role of the clinical leader is itself part of the NDU strategy, as is developing the clinical leadership potential of other team members. The clinical leader's role is demanding; many NDU's recognise this by appointing an administrative/secretarial post to assist them and the work of the NDU.

13. Empowerment of patients

The NDU seeks to involve those who receive nursing services, most importantly by sharing information. NDU nurses do not subscribe to the traditional professional view – of elites having power over others. Rather, knowledge is freely shared so that patients can make real choices in health care. Thus, many practices in the NDU will have a specific goal of patient empowerment – such as the support of patients' committees, advocacy schemes, providing access to health care records, creating 'user friendly' complaints procedures, self-medication programmes and so on.

14. Partnership in care

The NDU team not only work collaboratively with each other, they also develop models of practice which encourage shared caring and patient empowerment. Thus methods of organising care (such as primary nursing) which promote a one-to-one nurse/patient relationship and clearly delineate nursing responsibilities, are preferred. Nursing activities are organised to encourage patient/other carer participation in care, while recognising the many varied responses which patients may make along the dependence–independence continuum.

15. Patient-centred care

The NDU seeks to develop nurses in order to develop nursing. All the NDU's projects focus on the improvement of patient care, and it is the patient who holds the pivotal place in the NDU's activities. Every facet of the NDU is tested against this fundamental theme. It challenges all aspects of the way care is organised. Are routines appropriate to patients' needs? Is the allocation of nurses to patients organised most effectively? How does developing the nurse help the patient? By continuously questioning everything about its practice, the NDU helps build a climate of creativity in nursing, which ensures the NDU focus remains clearly on patient care, and not upon the completion of projects or NDU status as ends in themselves.

16. Involvement of other carers

The NDU team work collaboratively with other members of the multi-disciplinary team and others, such as relatives, who are involved in patient care. Strategies are developed, for example, to involve relatives in care where appropriate for them. Learning opportunities, project work, research findings and so on are shared with the multidisciplinary team. Indeed, the NDU may spark off innovations in other disciplines and many nursing projects may be open to collaborative work.

17. Equality in caring

The NDU is firmly committed to producing equity and equality in care for patients and other carers – regardless of age, sex, beliefs, culture or nationality. It is also committed to equal opportunities for its staff – in employment, learning and so on. The NDU shows its commitment to these in its policy documents, philosophy and practices. A review programme exists to ensure that these aspects can be maintained and acted upon if failings occur.

18. Organisational support

The NDU is formally supported by the organisation in which it is sited. Those with executive authority have explicitly committed themselves to support the NDU (in writing). This helps to legitimise the work of the NDU, raise its profile and encourages a dialogue with management. All of these thus reduce potential conflicts and help nursing developments take place in a secure climate of organisational commitment. Manager, clinical staff and other interested persons (e.g. patients' representatives, finance officer, medical staff, etc.) are included in an advisory board which meets regularly to generate support and help guide the NDU along its objectives.

19. Financial resources

The NDU has its own budget as with any other unit of the organisation in which it is sited. It may develop an income generation strategy to seek research monies, fund further staff development and generally expand its work. Resources for staffing, equipment and so on are agreed and explicit. Resources earmarked for education and development work are controlled by the NDU itself. The clinical leader has a pivotal role to play in the control and allocation of resources. Where specific funds are earmarked for nursing development projects, these are exclusively controlled by the NDU team. The NDU may actively seek further resources for its work.

20. Staff development

An extensive programme of staff development is an essential policy of the NDU. This has a number of features:

- The programme is demand-led by the nursing team and a strategy agreed.
- The opportunities for development are wide ranging e.g. attendance at courses and conferences, formal educational programmes, open learning facilities, study groups, project work, role modelling,

appraisal systems, exchange schemes, clinical supervision, reflective practice, etc., etc. Many options are available.
- Links are formed with a recognised educational institution to provide support; such as a college of nursing, university department, etc.

Underpinning the development is the recognition of its nature. The NDU does not just provide learning about nursing practice, but adopts strategies to empower the nurse. These include programmes to develop personal growth, autonomy, awareness and assertiveness. The NDU empowers nurses by equipping them with knowledge and skill in nursing as well as knowledge of themselves.

21. Dissemination

A strategy for disseminating the work of the NDU is necessary, otherwise there is a risk that any improvements remain focused on the NDU and are not transmitted to help nurses and patients elsewhere. This strategy will incorporate many aspects of outreach work according to local circumstances, for example:

- regular open days
- visitors' programmes and study days
- circulation of written reports
- team members teaching elsewhere, speaking at conferences, etc.
- networking with other NDUs, professional groups, etc.
- publishing papers
- circulating reports.

Many options are available. The important issue is that the NDU opens itself up to scrutiny and commits itself to sharing its work in many ways so that others may learn from its experiences, as Fig. 5.2 suggests.

NDUs also tend to increase in number. Some nurses not only apply individual practices developed in the NDU, but seek to create an NDU in their own area (Fig. 5.3).

Thus, to some extent, the nature of the organisation in which the NDU is set is less important than the support it receives and the quality of work the nurses undertake. NDUs are built on the assumption that, in time, ideas will spread. No matter what the barriers are, eventually innovations are able to transcend these. That is not to say the NDU exerts influence or pressure on others to accept and copy slavishly what it has done. Rather it holds it up to critical scrutiny so that others can learn from its experiences and make choices between which practices may be followed and which rejected.

If the UK example is considered, NDUs have contributed to innovations throughout the health care system (e.g. the spread of primary

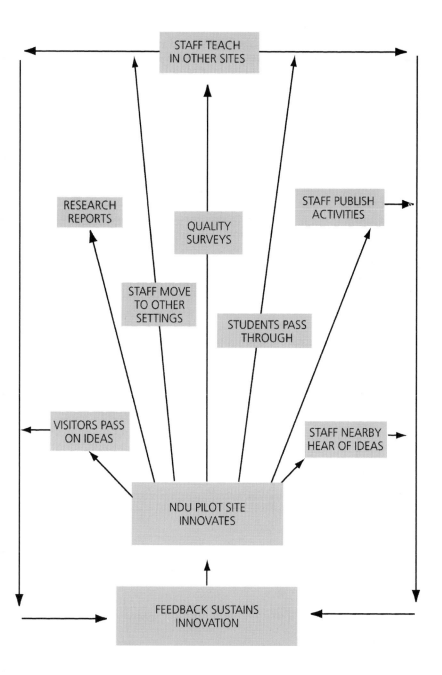

Figure 5.2 Dissemination: NDUs influence other settings

nursing) while at the same time increasing their own numbers. Thus the concept of the NDU has itself generated interest and replication, while the innovations planned in them have spread to far more places than the NDUs themselves.

Many NDUs have been self-financing with no additional resources (as in Tameside's example). However, the work of the King's Fund Programme and its allocation of government-funded grants, suggests

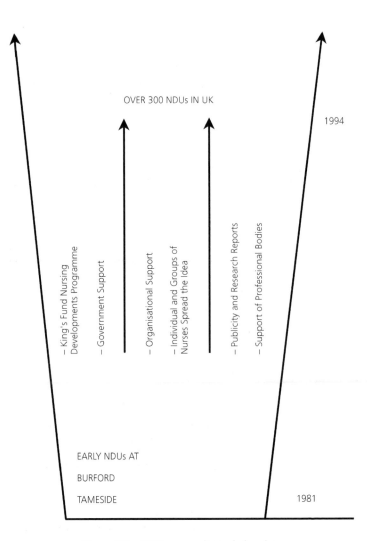

OVER 300 NDUs IN UK

1994

– King's Fund Nursing
Developments Programme

– Government Support

– Organisational Support

– Individual and Groups of
Nurses Spread the Idea

– Publicity and Research Reports

– Support of Professional Bodies

EARLY NDUs AT

BURFORD

TAMESIDE

1981

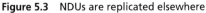

Figure 5.3   NDUs are replicated elsewhere

that progress can be much more rapid with an injection of pump priming and project money.

From Fig. 5.3 it can be seen that the number of UK NDUs has increased dramatically. In Europe, a similar process is under way. The European Nursing Development Agency (TENDA), for example, is now working with 11 sites which are all at varying stages of becoming NDUs. The American 'Project Hope' is funding similar ventures and the WHO (Nursing and Midwifery) European programme is stimulating further similar developments in the field. The general principles of the NDU are universal (managing change, teamwork, innovation in practice, etc.), but their application will vary from country to country.

22. Evaluation

An extensive programme of evaluation is devised. Once again this has many dimensions. The strategy will include different options appropriate to different settings, but all NDUs will tend to apply:

- setting and monitoring standards of care
- documenting the history of the NDU as it unfolds (e.g. some staff may agree to keep diaries of events)
- all projects/research include an evaluation element
- gathering baseline data before the NDU is set up and reviewing and comparing these later
- regular review meetings covering all aspects of the NDU's practices, documents, etc.
- defining an on-going quality assurance strategy (for example in Appendix 5.3). This includes the evaluation of care which elicits responses from patients, staff and others
- evaluation results are made openly available e.g. through circulated reports, journal papers, etc.
- regular and annual reports produced and circulated.

CASE STUDY

Comparison of Principles 1–22 with the example of the Tameside NDU

1   Recognised in the original work done on the philosophy of nursing by the staff. Many subsequent projects (e.g. changing the management climate, applying primary nursing, piloting nursing beds, etc.) sought to explore the organisation of care to facilitate the application of nursing as a therapy. Skill mix changed to increase number of qualified staff.

2   The NDU was a self-managed unit. Nursing roles were defined. The dependent–interdependent–independent relationship to medicine clarified. Staff development work sought to reinforce this. Nursing projects led by nurses.

CASE STUDY – *Contd*

3   Based in a clinical setting (the care of older people with acute health problems). The NDU was creatéd and led by clinical nurses.

4   Began on one ward, but expanded over ten years, with agreement of others, to include nine wards and a day hospital. Other nearby units affiliated to it, contributed to knowledge and spread of NDUs nationwide.

5   Change agent appointed and 'bottom-up' change strategy used (based on the work of Ottoway, Lewin and Turrill). Clinical staff at ward level defined and controlled the changes. Managers and educators acted as facilitators. Programme of changes documented. Changes continued, new ideas constantly being introduced. The NDU itself changed in nature, structure and goals.

6   Nursing culture emerged which broke away from the old ritualised institutionalised mould, generating commitment to change and new interests in nursing.

7   Philosophy documented and reviewed every two years. Used to underpin work on standards, the nursing model objectives for change, etc. Used in staff recruitment, team building. Available to public.

8   Developed and documented over a four-year period. Continues to evolve.

9   Multiplicity of projects pursued with staff involved at all levels e.g. primary nursing, self-medication, out of uniform trials, pet therapy, complementary therapies, standard setting, patient access to nursing records, designing patient information books, changing ward routines, patient teaching plans, care planning system, etc. Some staff led projects, others supported them. Funding pursued to support some projects. Planning and evaluation carried out.

10 New roles for nursing explored – primary nursing, continence adviser, clinical specialists, consultant nurse, ethnic needs worker, reminiscence therapist, etc. Practices developed to include some work previously undertaken by doctors, appropriate roles of support workers identified (e.g. ward clerks), expansion of nursing role. Skill mix changed to increase proportions of qualified staff.

11 Variety of projects pursued, from small scale ones, to others undertaken as part of course fulfilment – MSc and PhD theses. Staff attended ENB research courses. Clinical specialists and consultant had research advisory roles. Research forum formed. Journals purchased. Research funds sought and used.

12 Clinical leader appointed (initially jointly appointed nurse-tutor and charge nurse, later to become consultant nurse). Each ward identified its own clinical leader with further development. Resources controlled by NDU team. Development plans included for other team members.

13 Information-sharing policy developed, including access to nursing records, standards of care, information centres, information books, etc. Patients' committees formed. Advice of external agents sought (e.g. Age Concern).

14 Primary nurses work as partners with patients. Code of behaviour among team agreed and documented. Multidisciplinary team involved in many

CASE STUDY – *Contd*

aspects of the NDU's activities – including social occasions, shared learning opportunities, joint project work, etc.

15 Total realignment of clinical activity took place to break the institutional mould and produce a more patient-centred climate. Modification to environment (improvements to buildings; decor, furniture, etc.) made. Greater emphasis on individual need and less on ward routines and rituals, e.g. openness of visiting times, removal of fixed 'bedtimes', access to information, etc.

16 Collaborative work undertaken in many areas. Age Concern representatives invited to form advocacy scheme. Guidelines for relatives' participation in care agreed. Relative/patient teaching plans developed. Ward routines re-organised to permit maximum participation (e.g. removal of rigid visiting times).

17 Included in ward philosophy and monitored through evaluation process. Ethnic specialist appointed. Authority equal opportunities regulations applied and monitored.

18 Agreed (in writing) after negotiation at all levels. One manager had specific remit to support the NDU. NDU trustees and advisory board created.

19 Budget allocation defined. Ward budgets created. Trust funds set up. Income generation plan put into action (e.g. study days, visitors' fees, sale of information packs and other items, consultancy fees charged, etc., etc.).

20 Wide-ranging strategy agreed. Staff offered off-site courses and conferences, from short seminars to full-time degree programmes. Courses designed for all grades of staff whether nursing auxiliaries or qualified staff. Special courses for clinical leaders led by psychotherapist, including residential weekend. Therapist also undertook personal growth and awareness courses for other staff. On-site library developed. Open learning packages provided. Staff teaching and careers counselling roles identified (e.g. consultant nurse and clinical specialists). Many on-site workshops and study programmes devised. Clinical supervision and reflective practice introduced. Support derived from links with a university department of nursing and the local college of nursing, technical college and polytechnic. International exchange schemes developed.

21 Enormous amount of publicity generated (over 500 publications and press reports in ten years). Radio and TV contributions. Staff delivered many conference papers, led workshops, etc. NDU visitors' days set up. Information packs prepared. Longer placements offered to students, visitors, etc. Staff networked with others in the speciality, lobbied MPs, attended local support groups and so on. Many staff active in professional organisations (e.g. RCN).

22 NDU history evaluated by independent researcher. Nursing standards set. Quality assurance strategy developed. Quality assurance nurse appointed. All projects evaluated. Patients, staff, visitors' questionnaires and interview schedules devised. Baseline data gathered and compared annually (bed occupancy, pressure sore rates, incontinence levels, death rates, readmission rates, patient satisfaction comments, patient complaints, staff leavers surveys, etc.). Results published. Annual report produced.

More details are contained in Mary Black's (1991) independent research.

Summary

The focus of NDUs is the recognition that to develop nursing, it is also necessary to develop nurses. Nurses are the largest number of health care workers, therefore, any improvements they can bring can have a major impact on health care overall, probably more than introducing change in any other single discipline.

An NDU demonstrates that caring need not cost more and indeed, by recruiting and retaining well motivated and skilful staff, it can contain costs far better than settings that do not meet the standards of the NDU. The aspirations and aims of NDUs seem to have many common elements. What drives them above all is a commitment to changing nursing practice and a shared vision of the future – a better future for both patients and nurses. NDUs do not claim to be centres of excellence – but they do aspire to them.

When creating an NDU, however, the question must first be asked, why do we want one? The potential benefits to patients and nurses are not without problems. Some managers, doctors and others may find it more difficult to cope with more assertive, knowledgeable and empowered nurses. They may make greater demands for knowledge, education and the freedom to practise. Many nurses may respond to the NDU with praise, support and a willingness to learn from it, but others may display jealousy, hostility, a refusal to accept its ideas – the common responses when we fear change or find it difficult to acknowledge the work of leaders and pioneers. Organisational support, too, can have its problems. For example, the NHSME Objectives (1993) stated that 'the spread of Nursing Development Units and the good practice they foster, should be encouraged'. Thus, good intentions of organisational support may lead to increased pressure on nurses to create NDUs by management 'top-down' edict, rather than allow gradual 'bottom-up' growth from clinical level.

Furthermore, developing nurses has implications beyond the NDU site. There is a knock-on effect outside the profession. Empowered and developed nurses may question their personal and domestic lives and the social *status quo*.

NDUs can also contribute to the development of the service as a whole and to other disciplines. When nurses are clear about their own value and vision, they are in a better position to work collaboratively. Already in the UK, more general 'Practice Development Units' (Williams *et al.*, 1993) are emerging, partly in response to demands for 'inclusiveness' by others in the multidisciplinary team and partly to overcome changes of elitism (see also Chapter 7, page 154 relating to 'tall poppies'). Once again, they are not a panacea, but yet another option in the jigsaw puzzle of service development. The more options that can be used, the greater the potential benefits to patient care.

The NDU is more than a fixed ward, department or locality – these serve only to provide the clinical focus for its activities. The NDU is the people who work in it, what they do, how they relate to each other and their clients and how they change themselves and their practices.

Some NDUs are more mature than others and not all will meet the criteria listed in this text. For some, meeting all will be impossible (e.g. in some European countries, a link with a college or university department may not be possible as these may not exist locally). Many NDUs will be at different levels of attainment of the principles, but they share a commitment to pursue them. It is important to remember that the concept is not a nursing *developed* unit but a nursing *development* unit. The latter relates to the nature of the NDU as an evolving entity, not fixed and having totally achieved all its goals as the former would imply. In addition, there is no guarantee that the NDU will be a permanent feature – they tend to come and go as needs are fulfilled, or as support is lost because of their challenging nature (Naish, 1997). Being clear about objectives, survival tactics and dissemination strategies is essential to their continued progress.

NDUs are one means among many that change can be wrought in nursing practice. There are other options which may be more appropriate in different settings. They are not panaceas. They will not cure nursing's ills overnight. However, they do have a crucial role to play in liberating nursing to develop creative, compassionate caring, to think about, explore, value and enjoy nursing.

In the future, when all nurses practise excellent, thoughtful, creative, high quality nursing (and are supported in all ways to do so), NDUs may be redundant – for then every setting will accept that change is a way of life and the support of nurses to achieve perfection will have been accomplished. Even so, there will probably always be a need for centres of clinical nursing to research and explore its boundaries. Meanwhile, NDUs have a role to play – they may not yet embody perfection in nursing, but they do aim for it and offer hope and encouragement to others to do likewise.

References

Bamber, T., Johnson, M.L., Purdy, E. and Wright, S.G. 1989 The Tameside experience. *Nursing Standard* **22**(3), 26.

Benner, P. 1984 *From novice to expert.* Addison Wesley, London.

Black, G. 1992 *Nursing development units – work in progress.* King's Fund, London.

Black, M. 1993 *The growth of the Tameside nursing development unit.* King's Fund Centre, London.

Christian, S. and Redfern, S. 1996 Three years on: how NDUs are meeting the challenge. *Nursing Times* **92**(47) 35–37.

Cole, A. and Vaughan, B. 1994 *Reflections three years on.* King's Fund, London.

Dalley, G. 1988 *Ideologies of caring – rethinking the community and collectivism.* Macmillan, London.

Freeman, R. 1996 *How to become a Nursing Development* Unit. King's Fund, London.

Kitson, A. 1988 On the concept of nursing care. In: Fairbairn, G. and Fairbairn, S. (Eds), *Ethical issues in caring.* Gower, Aldershot.

MacMahon, R. and Pearson, A. 1991 *Nursing as therapy.* Chapman & Hall, London.

Mangan, P. 1992 Where from here? *Nursing Times* **88**(50), 34–35.

Naish, J. 1997 A lost opportunity. *Nursing Standard* **11**(25) 17.

National Health Service Management Executive 1993 *Objectives 1993–94.* NHSME, Leeds.

Pearson, A. 1983 *The clinical nursing unit.* Heinemann, London.

Pearson, A. (Ed.) 1988 *Primary nursing.* Croom Helm, London.

Pearson, A. 1992 *Nursing at Burford, a story of change.* Scutari, Harrow.

Pearson, A., Punton, S. and Durand, I. 1992 *Nursing beds – an evaluation of the effects of therapeutic nursing.* Scutari, Harrow.

Punton, S. 1989 The Oxford experience. *Nursing Standard* **22**(3), 27–28.

Purdy, E., Wright, S.G. and Johnson, M.L.J. 1988 Change for the better. *Nursing Times* **84**(38) 34–36.

Salvage, J. 1988 Nursing developments. *Nursing Standard* **22**(3), 25.

Salvage, J. and Wright, S.G. 1995 *Nursing Development Units.* Scutari, Harrow.

Turner-Shaw, J. and Bosanquet, N. 1993 *A way to develop nurses and nursing.* King's Fund Centre, London.

Vaughan, B. 1992 The pursuit of excellence. *Nursing Times* **88**(31), 26–28.

Williams, C., Lee, D. and Lowry, M. 1993 Practice development units: the next step? *Nursing Standard* **8**(11), 25–29.

Wright, S.G. 1987a *Building and using a model of nursing.* Arnold, London.

Wright, S.G. 1987b *My patient, my nurse: the practice of primary nursing.* Scutari, Harrow.

Wright, S.G. 1988 Developing nursing: the contribution to quality. *International Journal of Health Care Quality Assurance* **1**(1), 12–15.

Wright, S.G. 1989 *Changing nursing practice.* Arnold, London.

Wright, S.G. 1989 Defining the NDU. *Nursing Standard* **4**(7), 29–31.

Wright, S.G. 1992 Exporting excellence. *Nursing Times* **88**(39), 40–42.

Appendix 5.1

Example of a nursing philosophy – The Tameside NDU (1990)

It is our belief that the purpose of the Care of the Elderly Nursing Development Unit is to meet the goals of nursing as a functioning unit of the nursing service of the Health Authority.

We believe that each patient is an individual with the right to appropriate skilled nursing to meet his/her needs, and to have real freedom of choice in his/her care. The nursing service provided should be personal and responsive to the patient as a person, demonstrating respect for his/her integrity, individuality and uniqueness. The patient has a right to a knowledge and understanding of his/her condition and problems to enable him/her to make realistic choices, and to be given help and information so that he/she can understand and accept the treatment and care needed. These rights extend to all patients regardless of age, sex, race or creed and can be summarised thus:

The patient has the right to:

1 Skilled care, by all members of the hospital team, to meet his/her needs.

2 Know how and why he/she is being treated and what is being done to help him/her and what alternatives are available.

3 Be given enough information and skill to be as independent as possible.

4 Have choice in his/her care and be given enough knowledge so that he/she can make rational decisions.

5 Be treated as an individual and accorded respect, dignity and equal quality of care, regardless of age, sex, religion, race or beliefs.

6 Have total support, with the nurse and other members of the team acting on his/her behalf and in his/her best interests, when he/she is unable to make such choices for himself/herself.

We believe each ageing person to be a whole and unique person with a right to his/her own lifestyle in his/her own environment, and made up of complex and interdependent physical, social and psychological and spiritual needs. These contribute to make up the total person for whom ageing is a normal process in the continuum of human life.

We therefore believe that ageing is not necessarily synonymous with illness and the old person is entitled to a sense of learning, achievement and development throughout the ageing years. The old person has the right to be as healthy and happy as is possible in old age. To this end, it is the aim of nursing to work in partnership with him/her, to help relatives and other carers to maintain and improve health, and to help with investigation, correct diagnosis, treatment and rehabilitation when illness occurs. Nursing care must therefore be organised in such a way that enables a therapeutic relationship to exist between nurse, patient and other carers. It is our belief that the system known as primary nursing best facilitates this. The patient has the right to skilled nursing working in the multidisciplinary team, which will help him/her to be as independent as possible, to maintain dignity and foster a sense of identity either in the promotion of health and recovery, or assisting to achieve a peaceful and painfree death.

We believe that to achieve these ideals the Nursing Development Unit must foster the following main aims:

1 The unit is to be developed and maintained at a level where all activities are focused on the central function of meeting the individual needs of each individual patient.

2 Within this patient-orientated setting, it is recognised that the needs of all nurses to develop their knowledge and expertise must also be met. To this end a climate is to be nurtured which encourages the growth of learning and researching in parallel with that of patient care.

3 It is further held that the production of such an environment, where patient and personal needs are given paramount attention, is best fostered in an atmosphere where the staff adopt a positive attitude to the patients and each other. Thus it is essential that all staff of whatever grade work together as a team in spirit of cooperation, to maintain coordination of patient care and liaison with other hospital departments, and community staff, relatives and other carers.

4 Interpersonal relationships of a positive nature are considered to be significant in this climate, and are best encouraged by avoiding rigid authoritarianism based on rank. Decisions are to be made in a state of mutual respect and maximum consultation among staff wherever possible, and each trained nurse is accountable for the care he/she gives according to the United Kingdom Central Council for Nurses, Midwives and Health Visitors Code of Professional Conduct.

5 The Nursing Development Unit shall support the evaluation of care and the assessing of its quality. Patients and other carers should be involved in this process.

To ensure that the values expressed in this philosophy are put into practice, nurses in the Nursing Development Unit will pursue the following goals:

1   To enhance the development and status of Nursing the Elderly as a speciality in its own right.

2   To promote excellence in nursing practice with the elderly.

3   To continue the development of a nursing model for the elderly, based on partnership with patients, relatives and other carers.

4   To promote nursing practices which produce individualised nursing, including the development of primary nursing.

5   To provide a climate for nursing the elderly in which learning and ideas flourish, in which research is conducted and findings applied and in which our knowledge and experiences are disseminated to other nurses.

6   To motivate nurses to remain in the Unit and the speciality by providing professional development for all, with careers advice, educational plans and financial assistance.

7   To provide opportunities for nurses who have left to return to nursing, and to develop excellence in their practice and commitment to remaining in nursing.

8   To develop clinical nursing roles which permit those nurses prepared to commit themselves to the Unit and the speciality to enhance both their status and remuneration, while at the same time remaining in direct patient care.

9   To identify the desired standards of nursing care required by the elderly and to test, through the development of a variety of quality assurance methods, that these standards are being achieved.

10   To promote the full contribution of nursing to the multidisciplinary team to produce high standards of care for the elderly.

Appendix 5.2

The Nursing Development Unit – our nursing model (Tameside NDU example)

1   Nursing models are ways of thinking about and describing nursing, and help us make decisions about how best to organise care, e.g. if our approach is underpinned by partnership, then do we give patients access to information? Do we organise the ward using team nursing, task allocation, patient allocation or primary nursing?

2   Our nursing model is not just a theoretical model, it is a model in *practice*. It was created and developed by nurses *in* practice, and is

relevant to nursing care throughout the unit, 24 hours a day. Details have been well published (Wright, 1986). Our nursing model can most easily be identified by what we do. It is theory translated into practice and sometimes what we do is innovative and adds to nursing theory:

Practice

sharing information with patients / relatives / others
access to notes
access to other written information, complaints procedures, etc.
setting standards
patient / relative participation in care
care plans based on activities of living
open visiting
complementary therapies
primary nursing
reminiscence and pet therapy
mealtimes with patients
non-uniform wards
nurse-managed beds
self-medication, etc.

Management

quality assurance strategy
support for nursing development appraisal
counselling
provision of resources
supportive climate
developing new nursing roles
clinical support team

Education

staff development for all
developing skills to match the model
international exchange
clinical specialist roles
library, learning resources
development bursary

Research

support for finding out
seeking funds
writing up experiences / findings
small scale projects
NDU evaluation
etc., etc.

3 Our model has its origins in the initial development ward (ward 22) in 1981.

4 It is based on the unit's philosophy of nursing (see separate document) espousing key concepts of:

patients' and nurses' rights
partnership
problem-solving
advocacy
nursing as a therapy
holism
patient-centred practice
research-based practice
quality assurance and evaluation of practice
staff development.

5 The model has developed over time and is still changing as new ideas are tested and implemented, and outmoded ones discarded.

6 The model is not fixed, but dynamic and open to changes.

7 The unit philosophy acts as a foundation for individual ward philosophies.

8 Some concepts built into the model have been adapted from existing theoretical models e.g. self-care (Orem, 1980), activities of living (Henderson, 1966; Roper *et al.*, 1983). Both are used in the problem-solving phase.

9 Thus our nursing model is not just a theory, it is something that happens in practice. The NDU *is* a nursing model in action.

References to Appendix 5.2

Henderson, V. 1966 *The nature of nursing*. Macmillan, New York.
Orem, D.E. 1980 *Nursing – concepts of practice*. McGrower-Hills, New York.
Roper, N., Logan, W. and Tierney, A. 1983 *Using a model of nursing*. Churchill Livingstone, Edinburgh.
Wright, S.G. 1986 *Building and using a model of nursing*. Arnold, London.

Appendix 5.3

Quality in Nursing – Example of the Nursing Development Unit Model (1991)

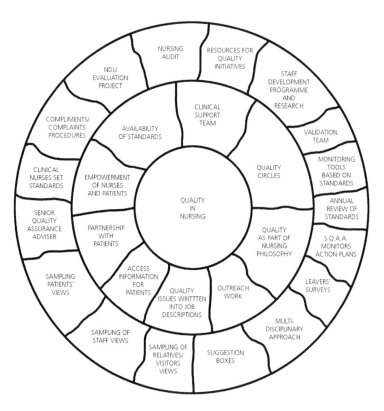

Figure 5.4 NDU model

Nurses at clinical level set and monitor nursing standards. It is fundamental to the approach of the NDU that a 'bottom-up' approach is used to ensure that standards are devised, written and accepted by nurses in practice.

A Senior Quality Assurance Adviser (SQAA) is in post to facilitate and coordinate the development of specific quality initiatives, and to monitor the achievement of nursing standards.

Annual random sampling of patients' views is conducted using questionnaires and interviews by the SQAA. Results are fed back to the clinical staff and management for action.

Staff views are sought annually by questionnaire and interview by the SQAA, and results are fed back to clinical staff and management for action.

Annual random sampling of relatives'/visitors' views is also conducted by questionnaires and results are fed back to clinical staff and management for action.

Suggestion boxes, with instructions in their use and with the necessary equipment provided, are situated at strategic points on the unit. These are checked weekly by the SQAA and dealt with according to an agreed protocol.

All nursing quality initiatives are focused on producing excellence in nursing practice.

Nursing quality initiatives do not take place in isolation, but are part of an overall model incorporating a multidisciplinary quality assurance approach.

Quality and standards responsibilities are clearly identified in every nurse's job description.

Annual staff appraisal and performance review includes an assessment of each member of staff's contribution to the quality of nursing care, acknowledges a positive contribution and sets action plans to remedy needs for further development.

Leavers' surveys among nursing staff are conducted by the SQAA to assess reasons for leaving, identify weaknesses in the organisation and suggest plans for further action.

A validation team which includes both staff and members of the public, reviews the nursing standards every year (see separate document). It makes recommendations for action and reviews achievements.

The SQAA monitors the application and outcomes of all development and action plans.

The NDU shares its standards and other quality initiatives with other members of the multidisciplinary team, with other sectors of the health authority, and with the nursing profession as a whole.

The clinical teams review their standards annually, make adjustments, and write new ones.

Monitoring tools, e.g. questionnaires/interview schedules, are based on the documented nursing standards.

Quality assurance is an integral part of the NDU philosophy and actions.

A comprehensive staff development programme is continually under way with opportunities for all levels of nursing staff and with an inclusion of quality assurance issues. The aim is to equip all staff with awareness of skills to contribute to their active role in quality promotion.

Quality circle activities are facilitated by the SQAA, and results of their deliberations are formulated into action plans supported by management.

A clinical support team of managers and nurse specialists is in existence to provide support to nursing staff in achieving standards, personal development and resources.

Patients/relatives/visitors are given full access to information about care, what standard is being achieved, how to present comments, compliments and complaints, and so on. Information books, copies of standards, etc. are available to patients and other carers, on the wards, local libraries, GP clinics, etc.

The philosophy and approach of the unit promotes sharing of information and a spirit of partnership between professionals and consumers.

Nursing standards and the results of monitoring are made available to the public and to the Community Health Council (CHC) as well as the usual channels in the health authority.

Key nurses in the unit contribute to the development of nursing standards and quality initiatives at local, regional and national level.

A nursing audit is conducted by the SQAA in each ward/department every other year. Acknowledgement for achievements is given. Action plans for improvement are drawn up. Results and recommendations are made available to clinical staff and managers.

Nurses in key posts contribute to multidisciplinary standard setting and monitoring.

The unit funds and resources quality initiatives, action plans and quality assurance tools and their use.

The NDU funds staff development and research projects.

6 Studies in change

Donna Davenport, Sue Pearce and Helena Kearsley

A vision without a task is but a dream. A task without a vision is drudgery. A vision and a task are the hope of the world.

A carving from a church in Sussex

The following studies were produced by three students following a clinical leadership programme at Central Manchester College of Nursing and Midwifery. Each describes the application of their clinical leadership skills to the process of managing change. They illuminate the complexity, joys and frustrations of being involved in change, and also show us how it is not just 'the system' which changes, but how it changes us as well.

STRUGGLING FOR CHANGE
Donna Davenport

> The ENP and *The scope of professional practice*
>
> Strategies for change
>
> My role as clinical leader
>
> Conclusion

The Emergency Nurse Practitioner (ENP) role was introduced into the Accident and Emergency (A & E) department where I worked in December 1994. Funding was made available by the Trust to initiate this service and to address the issue of increasing numbers of new attendance over the previous two years and the additional increase in waiting times for non-urgent or minor injuries.

Whilst waiting times have been addressed in the Patient's Charter Standards (NHSME, 1992) long delays for patients presenting to A&E appear to continue. ENPs have been introduced to busy A&E departments as one solution, although this innovation is in need of further evaluation to gauge its effectiveness.

I am a Sister in an A&E department and have played an active role in the development of the ENP since its introduction, despite the role being initially imposed upon the nursing staff. Whilst there were obvious pressures on my manager and senior medical staff to introduce this role, much of the resistance by nurses evolved as a direct result of the change being imposed upon them (Aird and Sale, 1990). I therefore looked at other strategies for change in order to develop the role further to enhance nursing development and improve the quality of care for patients (Benne and Chin, 1985). It was envisaged, by using alternative strategies, resistance and conflict would be avoided and staff would come to feel ownership of the role and the change in its development.

'Ownership of the change process and its results must be the prerogative of those who are doing the work. By owning the change the staff will come to feel it is their decision and that their experience and ideas are important. It is recognised that people tend to cherish, care for and preserve those things which they themselves have created' (Wright, 1989). This has been demonstrated in the way the more senior nurses have undertaken the role enthusiastically, recognising the value of such innovation in nursing practice.

I have, through self-awareness, been able to recognise resistance within myself and have been encouraged to develop my assertiveness skills through this project and through reflective practice.

Throughout this study I will concentrate on my role as a clinical leader and change agent in encouraging and nurturing my staff to become more self-aware also, and to inspire them to develop both themselves and the role of the ENP.

Despite the fact that the ENP role has been medically led, defined and controlled within my department, with evaluation being based on numbers seen and medical assessment of documentation after the patient had been discharged, nurses have strived to ensure that they are autonomous practitioners accountable for their practice. This has often been difficult and I have often needed to utilise my skills as a clinical leader to support my peers and avoid conflict which may have been detrimental to the important aspect of teamwork (Walsh, 1995).

I will also demonstrate how *The scope of professional practice* (UKCC, 1992) has been invaluable in shaping the development of this role and will allow nurses to develop and critically analyse their own practice.

This study defines the role of the ENP and the observed problems within my department. I also identify my role as a change agent and discuss the skills I have acquired in order to develop personally and professionally.

Clear rationale will be identified and goals set in order to achieve outcomes. Leadership issues will be analysed throughout and evaluation will be undertaken through reflection which is recognised 'as an active process of exploration and discovery and aims to link theory to practice' (Schon, 1983).

I intend to employ the knowledge of leadership concepts and principles I have acquired whilst on the Clinical Leadership course at Central Manchester College of Nursing and Midwifery to evaluate both my 'progress' and the development of the ENP role in the future. This will take the form of qualitative as well as quantitative measures, as to date, evaluation has been quantitative and has therefore not allowed nurses to identify their own learning needs and professional development.

By raising self-awareness, critical incident analysis and the use of a reflective journal, I was able to encourage staff to question their practice and put forward reasoned arguments to their managers. This is particularly important within the present climate of the ever-changing Health Service, in which nurses' roles are constantly being questioned and at times 'there is a growing sense of powerlessness among nurses in decisions which seem to directly affect themselves and their patients' (Wright, 1996).

In a department like mine where there has also recently been the introduction of Health Care Support Workers, it is important that nurses do not 'do unto others as they have had done unto them' i.e. delegate unwanted roles or tasks which seem unimportant or 'basic'. There is a real danger within A&E that nurses will lose sight of what constitutes nursing. I often feel great concern to hear junior staff comments regarding what they consider 'basic' acts such as bathing someone or helping someone with a fractured hip onto a bedpan. I feel these acts require a whole range of skill and interpersonal expertise. As nurses are swept along with the idea that only the high-tech skills are important in A&E in order to save a patient's life, it seems questionable as to whose interest the nurse is serving, the medical staff or the patient.

As Wright states (1991a) 'the therapeutic nurse has a very clear idea of what constitutes nursing and recognises that those acts often dismissed as basic are actually complex, intricate and valuable elements in their own right. Without them the essence of nursing is lost'. As nurses in A&E, it is important to ensure we have a clear understanding of what our role is, otherwise we will have no argument when others try to define our role for us. One of the main problems with the ENP role at present is that as nurses not involved in the decision to implement the role of the ENP, we felt that the restricted protocols which we were given to work with consisted of rules governing as to what we could and could not do.

I will also discuss the importance of policies and protocols which are 'an agreement to a particular set of activities which assist health care workers to respond consistently in complex areas of clinical practice' (RCNA&E Association, 1994).

However, when imposed and followed without question protocols can act as barriers to innovative and individualised nursing practice. Staff within my department have identified that such rigid protocols have restricted their practice and autonomy. Further recommendations to develop these protocols together with developing individual practitioners' self-awareness and critical incident analysis will be given.

It is evident within the scope of this study that I will only be able to give a brief insight into my project as a whole. Therefore it focuses on four main aspects:

1 The present role of the ENP and identifying the problems.

2 My role as a clinical leader in addressing these and relating theory to practice.

3 Future development of the ENP role.

4 Recommendations for strategies to ensure professional development of the individual practitioners.

The ENP and *The scope of professional practice*

An ENP has been defined as 'an autonomous practitioner, able to assess, diagnose, treat and discharge patients without reference to a doctor but within pre-arranged guidelines (Sbiah, 1994). As an ENP I am able to practise in this way working within agreed protocols to provide care for patients attending with minor injuries.

'The domino effect of the ENP means that seriously ill patients are receiving the best possible care, whilst the ENP by the nature of their work, diagnose, treat and discharge those attending with certain minor injuries in offering them an ideal treatment path if they wish so' (Sbiah, 1994).

In practice, however, this has not occurred as the ENP has also been expected to work within his/her capacity as an A&E nurse and due to staffing levels has been called to also deal with more seriously ill patients, as often the ENP is one of the more senior, experienced nurses.

This causes immense problems as the nurse is continually changing roles within any given shift, from dealing with minor injuries to major life-threatening conditions.

The ENP involved is then criticised by medical staff for allowing a queue of minor injuries to develop. Nurses within the department then become hostile and feel under stress. I have encouraged staff to be able to justify their actions, set priorities and put forward sound arguments as to why this happens.

As a Sister in the A&E department, I was once criticised for being 'too emotional' when expressing concern regarding staffing levels. Whilst I initially felt angry and upset at this remark, I then went away and reflected upon my actions and approach to the problem and was able to learn a great deal about my self-awareness, which resulted in me changing my practice based on this critical incident. I also found that using a reflective journal allowed me to write down my feelings and frustrations and change them into a positive learning experience which would, in the future, enable me to become more effective in my practice and would allow me to develop coping strategies in the future (Johns, 1994).

Whilst the number of ENPs in the UK continues to grow, the volume and range of nurse practitioner work varies immensely. Studies have found that ENP roles have developed sporadically and without clear definitions, their roles vary throughout the UK and depending on whether the department is a major A&E department or a minor injuries unit (Read *et al.*, 1992; Beales and Baker, 1995; Rees and Kinnersley, 1996).

A pilot study attempted to compare assessment and treatment of patients with minor injuries by nurse practitioners or junior doctors, but its findings were unsubstantiated due to the small numbers of patients managed by nurse practitioners compared with the greater numbers managed by junior doctors (Read and George, 1994).

As this is the case within my department, I would argue that this situation has arisen because of too stringent protocols being enforced restricting nursing practice and not encompassing the scope of professional practice recommendations (UKCC, 1992). As Ashworth (1992) notes: 'There have always been nurses willing to take on new responsibilities and accept accountability even before it was explicitly required of all nurses in the UK'.

This is particularly the situation in A&E departments where junior doctors rotate every six months and often experienced A&E nurses are left to support and teach them. Junior doctors often recognise the expertise of A&E nurses and are aware of their own inexperience in dealing with such a diverse area of medicine.

There seems then to be some concern if junior doctors are given such freedom to treat patients in A&E with little or no experience when experienced, highly skilled nurses are expected to adhere to stringent protocols.

The scope of professional practice (UKCC, 1992) states that 'nurses, as professionally accountable practitioners, must be able to develop their practice in line with new developments'.

'Along with this freedom goes the responsibility to make conscious, deliberate decisions about what activities they take on, with consideration of the consequences and in particular the consequences for their patients' (Ashworth, 1988).

By imposing strict protocols upon nurses it is questionable as to whether we have moved on from extended roles at all. As Wright (1991b) states 'the most important consideration in the whole debate is whether or not the patient gets a better deal as a result, in terms of quality of care'.

Had this been the key consideration in implementing the ENP role in my department I feel this change would have been more successful. Instead the rationale given for this change was:

- to reduce doctors' hours
- to free doctors to treat more acutely ill
- to reduce doctors' workload
- funding was made available
- nurses were cheaper than doctors.

I would suggest that these reasons are in direct conflict to the nursing rationale for taking on this role, that is:

- *The scope of professional practice* encouraging autonomous nursing practice;
- to improve the quality of care for patients with minor injuries;
- to provide holistic care to patients i.e. the nurse sees the patient through their whole time in A&E assessing, treating, discharging whilst at the same time able to offer health education, accident prevention advice and also prescribe certain medication.

Strategies for change

Whilst some of these criteria may overlap, I would suggest that had the rationale behind introducing the ENP role been discussed and clarified at clinical level its introduction would have been much smoother. Such a strategy would have encouraged active participation by the nurses involved using a bottom-up approach (normative–re-educative) which is argued to be more successful (Benne and Chin, 1985).

This strategy identifies that individuals are constantly attempting to satisfy needs and is guided by habits, attitudes, values and socio-cultural norms. By re-educating staff and explaining and encouraging discussion, attitudes and behaviour should be altered. It is recognised that change is more likely to be accepted if those who are to be affected are actually involved in it (Driscoll, 1982).

As Moss-Kanter (1984) notes: 'By ensuring that all kinds of people at all levels have the opportunity to contribute to solving problems, an organisation establishes an innovating culture'.

Indeed some of the most successful companies adopt this approach which has a deeply ingrained philosophy that says 'Respect the individual, make people winners, let them stand out and treat people as adults' (Peters and Waterman, 1982).

As National Health Services have become Trusts, and more emphasis is placed upon efficiency and cost-effectiveness it would seem appropriate to look at their most expensive item, i.e. nurses and the important role they have to play within the culture of the Health Service.

Within any large organisation there will be people who are perceived to be 'difficult'. Change is often perceived as a threat and each department will have driving forces and resisting forces. The way I approach people, therefore, has a direct bearing on the level of success in implementing further change to the ENP role. It has been demonstrated that people will respond imaginatively and responsibly when given the freedom to act (Aird and Sale, 1990).

An innovating culture encourages the release of the natural creative drive and commitment by the people who are directly responsible for providing a service which genuinely responds to patient/client needs. This approach also prevents conflict and confrontation. Conflict is defined as: 'Closely related to power and political issues, it is inevitable and can be destructive or constructive. It may offer an individual personal gain, provide prestige to the winner, be an incentive for creativity and serve as a powerful motivator' (Kennedy, 1992).

Because of the sheer range of human differences it is difficult to 'please' everyone, but an understanding of why there is resistance and strategies to reduce this will go a long way in alleviating these problems. There are many reasons why people resist change and it is up to the change agent to recognise this. Resistance to change is a natural phenomenon, which needs to be recognised, understood and managed (Plant, 1987).

It is recognised that within any given population affected by change there will be a small number of 'innovators' who will welcome and accept the change almost immediately and a similar number of 'laggards' who will resist the change to the end and may never see the benefit of it. In between are the majority of the population who will fall broadly into two groups: those who are likely to adopt the change and those who will take longer and need more convincing (Stewart, 1994).

I have observed a whole range of behaviour since the introduction of the nurse practitioner, from all grades of staff. I firmly believe that much of the resistance and dissatisfaction with the role by individuals has been caused by lack of professional support and on-going training and development. Continuous evaluation and opportunity to address problems are vital if this resistance and dissatisfaction are to cease.

I feel certain that by encouraging staff to develop at their own individual pace, able to set their own objectives and openly discuss issues, these problems will be alleviated and, more importantly, the number of patients seen by nurse practitioners who feel comfortable but challenged by this role will increase.

I would suggest that motivation for change was already present within this role. Staff identified their dissatisfaction with the current status, were critical of the service they were delivering (feeling that it was only a token of what they could achieve) and voiced their opinions as to what needed to change.

So how could I hope to overcome these problems as a Sister in the A&E department who also practises as a nurse practitioner? We needed to have a shared vision. Until we had the opportunity to share our ideas, rather than work in isolation, we were not able to identify what is required in order for us to develop further. It is said that 'a shared vision can give drive and encouragement to each other throughout the difficult change process' (Broome, 1990).

With effective leadership and the use of a 'bottom-up' change strategy I was able to stimulate a sense of commitment, feeling of ownership and wholeheartedness in developing this role at practice level.

However, I had to acknowledge that this strategy would not be effective in all situations and throughout my project it was necessary to evaluate and re-evaluate the various stages. Evaluation of the change should be an on-going process and retrogression to former practices avoided. Whilst undertaking this change it was necessary to continue to provide the service in its present state.

It was possible, however, for staff to clearly see the benefit as their practice developed and learning took place through self-awareness and reflective practice.

My role as clinical leader

Rafferty's (1991) research has indicated that there is no clear consensus in nursing about what leadership is or who the leaders are. Indeed confusion remains as to the very nature of leadership as opposed to management. It is often suggested that less management and more leadership is needed in the Health Services to cope with the increasing complexity of services and the world surrounding the service (Broome, 1990).

In response to this, courses in clinical leadership have emerged to address the needs of nurses at clinical level to develop their role as leaders. The courses focus very much upon self-awareness and require in-depth exploration of 'who I am and what makes me tick', change management and assertiveness. Emphasis is placed on the belief that you cannot take care of others unless you take care of yourself.

As a basis on which to become aware of yourself, the course required students to undertake a Myers–Briggs Type Indicator Test

(Briggs and Myers, 1987). This test is based on the theory of personality types between people on four separate scales. Each scale represents two opposite preferences, one of which we normally like to choose or use in daily life. Our preferences for either end of each of these four scales can be translated into a set of insights into our relative strengths and areas for further growth and development, to maximise our potential and help us to appreciate ourselves and others.

My 'type' emerged as ESTJ (*see* Fig. 6.1). Reflecting on these attributes has enabled me to develop my leadership skills further and build upon areas requiring further development. In recognising my own strengths and weaknesses I feel comfortable but challenged in my role as an A&E Sister and as a nurse practitioner. In demonstrating my expertise and knowledge and sharing this with my colleagues I feel I am approachable and staff look to me as a good role model and leader. However, it is important that I am able to recognise when I need support and how and where to get it. An effective leader must be able to develop and grow as well as the people they are expected to lead.

Leadership is defined as 'the ability to identify a goal, come up with a strategy for achieving that goal and inspire your team to join you in putting that strategy into action' (Rafferty, 1991).

Within my department I identified my goal of improving the role of the nurse practitioner to benefit both staff and patients. I had already been approached by several members of staff with sound ideas and support for this project. By involving staff from the beginning its chances of long-term success were increased. It was important that the people who would be affected by the change should be involved whenever possible from the beginning.

It was envisaged that my 'allies' would help to move forward the more reluctant members of the team, whilst acknowledging that there will always be 'difficult' people within any organisation who may never see the benefits of any developments or change.

As a leader I needed to be aware of the impact such negativity can have upon a workforce and deal with this appropriately.

I discussed my project with my nurse manager and the A&E consultants, as it is imperative that their support was given if the proposal was to be a success.

To date the progress of my project has been slow due to the department being moved to a new purpose-built A&E unit. The impact of this change upon staff has been immense and I felt it inappropriate to introduce a further change which would mean more work and stress upon my colleagues. It is important as a leader to be aware of the workload of your team and avoid overload. As I have also been involved in developing health promotion/education, developing a formal document for telephone advice and re-writing the A&E

Sensing Types   Intuitive Types

ISTJ	**ISFJ**	**INFJ**	**INTJ**
Serious, quiet, earn success by concentration and thoroughness. Practical, orderly, matter-of-fact, logical, realistic, and dependable. See to it that everything is well organised. Take responsibility. Make up their own minds as to what should be accomplished and work toward it steadily, regardless of protests or distractions.	Quiet, friendly, responsible, and conscientious. Work devotedly to meet their obligations. Lend stability to any project or group. Thorough, painstaking, accurate. Their interests are usually not technical. Can be patient with necessary details. Loyal, considerate, perceptive, concerned with how other people feel.	Succeed by perseverance, originality, and desire to do whatever is needed or wanted. Put their best efforts into their work. Quietly forceful, conscientious, concerned for others. Respected for their firm principles. Likely to be honoured and followed for their clear convictions as to how best to serve the common good.	Usually have original minds and great drive for their own ideas and purposes. In their fields that appeal to them, they have a fine power to organise a job and carry it through with or without help. Sceptical, critical, independent, determined, sometimes stubborn. Must learn to yield less important points in order to win the most important.
ISTP	**ISFP**	**INFP**	**INTP**
Cool onlookers – quiet, reserved, observing and analysing life with detached curiosity and unexpected flashes of original humour. Usually interested in cause and effect, how and why mechanical things work, and in organising facts using logical principles.	Retiring, quietly friendly, sensitive, kind, modest about their abilities. Shun disagreements, do not force their opinions or values on others. Usually do not care to lead but are often loyal followers. Often relaxed about getting things done, because they enjoy the present moment and do not want to spoil it by undue haste or exertion.	Full of enthusiasms and loyalties, but seldom talk of these until they know you well. Care about learning, ideas, language, and independent projects of their own. Tend to undertake too much, then somehow get it done. Friendly, but often too absorbed in what they are doing to be sociable. Little concerned with possessions or physical surroundings.	Quiet and reserved. Especially enjoy theoretical or scientific pursuits. Like solving problems with logic and analysis. Usually interested in ideas, with little liking for parties or small talk. Tend to have sharply defined interests. Need careers where some strong interest can be used and useful.
ESTP	**ESFP**	**ENFP**	**ENTP**
Good at on-the-spot problem-solving. Do not worry, enjoy whatever comes along. Tend to like mechanical things and sports, with friends on the side. Adaptable, tolerant, generally conservative in values. Dislike long explanations. Are best with real things that can be worked, handled, taken apart, or put together.	Outgoing, easygoing, accepting, friendly, enjoy everything and make more fun for others by their enjoyment. Like sports and making things happen. Know what's going on and join in eagerly. Find remembering facts easier than mastering theories. Are best in situations that need sound common sense and practical ability with people as well as with things.	Warmly enthusiastic, high-spirited, ingenious, imaginative. Able to do almost anything that interests them. Quick with a solution for any difficulty and ready to help anyone with a problem. Often rely on their ability to improvise instead of preparing in advance. Can usually find compelling reasons for whatever they want.	Quick, ingenious, good at many things. Stimulating company, alert and outspoken. May argue for fun on either side of a question. Resourceful in solving new and challenging problems, but may neglect routine assignments. Apt to turn to one new interest after another. Skilful in finding logical reasons for what they want.
ESTJ	**ESFJ**	**ENFJ**	**ENTJ**
Practical realistic, matter-of-fact, with a natural head for business or mechanics. Not interested in subjects they see no use for, but can apply themselves when necessary. Like to organise and run activities. May make good administrators, especially if they remember to consider others' feelings and points of view.	Warm-hearted, talkative, popular, conscientious, born cooperators, active committee members. Need harmony and may be good at creating it. Always doing something nice for someone. Work best with encouragement and praise. Main interest is in things that directly and visibly affect people's lives.	Responsive and responsible. Generally feel real concern for what others think or want, and try to handle things with due regard for the other person's feelings. Can present a proposal or lead a group discussion with ease and tact. Sociable, popular, sympathetic. Responsive to praise and criticism.	Hearty, frank, decisive, leaders in activities. Usually good in anything that requires reasoning and intelligent talk, such as public speaking. Are usually well informed and enjoy adding to their fund of knowledge. May sometimes appear more positive and confident than their experience in an area warrants.

Introverts / Extroverts (left margin labels for Sensing Types)

Figure 6.1 Characteristics frequently associated with each type from Myers, I. and Briggs K.C. (1987)

department Philosophy of Care, it is evident that I had to give some areas of work more priority than others.

Stress is an inevitable part of any change process to some degree and needs to be recognised. Salvage (1988) notes that when nurses complain that they cannot cope, they are often held to blame, instead of examining the situation which has produced the failure to cope. By supporting staff through the change process, particularly a move to a new department, I feel they have coped admirably and have seen it as a challenge.

A support group has been formed including myself as the facilitator, and two members of the ENP team following discussions within the department. The very nature of A&E work is varied, diverse and practically orientated and, as such, lends itself to group discussion of practice (Castille, 1994).

At present peer group review work is undertaken by medical staff on a weekly basis within our department. It was felt that a similar programme should be available to nursing staff and would be a way of introducing nurses to the concept of reflective practice and critical incident analysis. Similar work in other departments has been demonstrated to be a success in providing a practical framework which could be applied to the clinical setting of the A&E department and benefit patient care (Castille, 1996).

A random selection of cards was chosen to stimulate group discussion regarding a particular case. Before, nursing staff had no way of evaluating their performance in relation to the ENP role which means that they had no opportunity to obtain feedback on their performance within this important role. By stimulating group discussion in a non-threatening environment it was envisaged that this situation would be resolved. By reflecting on the care given, standard of record keeping, ethical considerations and case management, this can lead to new understanding and appreciation which can be put to use in future experiences (Dewing, 1990).

The previous practice of senior medical staff randomly selecting nurse practitioner notes to evaluate care was non-productive and often the only discussion which took place was when care was deemed incorrect or inappropriate. Such an approach serves neither the nurse nor the patient in improving care, whereas reflective learning effects a deepening and enhancement of knowledge and skills. Reflection-on-action is encouraged by providing a stimulating learning environment and time to discuss problems and how such problems may be resolved to influence future care (Walker, 1996).

Each session would be documented by individuals and support group members in order to take back to the consultants and nurse manager any areas which could not be dealt with in the group, i.e. areas for further education and training.

The practice of documenting such discussions would also be beneficial for reflection purposes and as evidence of further development in line with post-registration education requirements (UKCC, 1990).

As nurse practitioners may be present whose cards were randomly selected, there was also an opportunity to put forward rationales as to why the outcome was good or bad or, more significantly, outside the boundaries of the set protocols. Again this gave the nurse the chance to put forward sound arguments in defence of his/her 'risk taking' (Wallace, 1996) which in turn may have implications for developing the nurse practitioner protocols. Reflection can be utilised by nurses in assisting them to identify routinised practice, make changes and internalise new values and attitudes (Jarvis, 1992).

As much of the work in A&E could be seen as task allocation with the role of the nurse as a passive deliverer of acute care based on a medical model, I envisaged that the changes in the development of nurse practitioners would greatly increase their autonomy within this role.

As staff came to see and feel the benefits of this exciting innovation, I felt the idea of reflection and critical thinking would lead to a natural progression and implementation of clinical supervision. This concept has been implemented with great success in areas of psychiatry, midwifery and care of the elderly (Kohner, 1994) and it seems patients and staff alike will benefit.

It is argued that clinical supervision is a major force in improving clinical standards, enhancing the quality of care and ensuring less strain and burnout in nursing staff by encouraging more self-awareness and self-expression (Faugier and Butterworth, 1992).

However, it is imperative that clinical supervision does not become yet another target or imposition from managers or academics upon those working in clinical practice (Butterworth, 1994). As a Sister in the A&E department I endeavoured to ensure that such an innovation was not imposed upon staff in this way so that it would be undertaken with wholeheartedness and commitment.

Clinical supervision must be implemented for the right reasons and should be separate from issues relating to pay, promotion or discipline, only then can a trusting relationship be fostered (Holt, 1995). In the past I have experienced how suspicion is aroused when managers introduce new concepts without clearly identifying the rationale behind them to the staff who will be directly participating in them.

Proctor (1991) suggests a tripartite approach to supervision:

- *Formative*
  Focuses on the educative process of developing the skills, understanding and abilities of the supervisee.

- *Restorative*
  Relies on support, exploring anxieties or critical incidents and allowing the supervisee to resolve stress.

- *Normative*
  The managerial aspect of supervision which provides a crucial 'quality control' element which is absolutely essential in all work with people.

The success of clinical supervision relies heavily upon how it is implemented and its perceived benefits to the department. As a Sister committed to ensuring staff development and support are available to all staff I have ensured I have worked closely with my manager to ensure my clinical expertise was utilised to the full in implementing this concept.

I feel that by gradually introducing the staff to this innovation in the form of peer group review they began to feel comfortable with clinical supervision on an individual basis. As someone who was in a senior position and had recently experienced the benefits and rewards of clinical supervision, at a particularly stressful time in my career, I can only advocate clinical supervision as a major development in the pursuit of nursing excellence.

It is not within the scope of this study to go into great depth regarding clinical supervision. However, it was necessary to demonstrate how my project could link well to the introduction of clinical supervision. In particular, it seems clinical supervision has the potential to address many of the problems related to nurses' work in such a difficult clinical area as Accident and Emergency.

Conclusion

The Clinical Leadership course has enabled me to become more self-aware both theoretically and in practice. I have developed further critical understanding of the main approaches used in the principles of management, change and leadership.

Within my practice I have been able to analyse and evaluate my own management and leadership skills which I hope have been demonstrated throughout my project.

I hope that through dissemination of my experiences in practice, and demonstration of the ability to use reflection as a learning process, my peers will clearly be able to see the benefits within my personal and professional development.

By encouraging and supporting my staff I hope to nurture a stimulating and rewarding environment. Working within the same clinical area I feel I have a sound understanding of the issues which cause concern and anxiety as well as those which staff feel are a challenge. I am often aware of the effect that saying 'thank you' at the end of a shift can have no matter how difficult or distressing it has been. Having an understanding of people and their behaviour can go a long way in bringing out the best in them.

Indeed, at a time when I felt I could not cope, reflection allowed me to express my feelings and analyse the incident in a positive way to determine what I had actually done within the situation.

My philosophy when things go wrong is now, in the words of Jeffers (1991), 'I'm not a failure because I didn't succeed; I'm a success because I tried' which I feel together with this course has allowed me to develop both personally and professionally to benefit both my team and the patients we are striving to care for.

References

Aird, B. and Sale, M. 1990 Agents of change. *Nursing Times* **86**(10), 43–46.

Ashworth, P. 1988 Boundaries of nursing. Editorial. *Intensive and Critical Care Nursing* 4(3), 93–94.

Ashworth, P. 1992 The scope of professional practice. Editorial. *Intensive and Critical Care Nursing* 8, 193.

Beales, J. and Baker, B. 1995 Minor injuries unit: expanding the scope of accident and emergency provision. *Accident and Emergency Nursing* **3**, 65–67.

Benne, K.D. and Chin, R. 1985 General strategies for effecting changes in human systems. *The Planning of Change*. C.B.S. College Publications, London, 1995.

Broome, A.K. 1990 *Managing change: essentials of nursing management.* Macmillan Education, London.

Butterworth, T. 1994 Preparing to take on clinical supervision. *Nursing Standard* 8(52), 32–34.

Castille, K. 1994 The role of the A&E nurse. Unpublished Thesis. Manchester Metropolitan University, Manchester.

Castille, K. 1996 Clinical supervision from rhetoric to Accident & Emergency practice. *Accident & Emergency Nursing* 4(1), 2–4.

Dewing, J. 1990 Reflective practice. *Senior Nurse* **10**(10), 26–28.

Driscoll, S. 1982 Nurses and the change process. *New Zealand Nursing Journal* **75**(2), 3–4.

Faugier, J. and Butterworth, T. 1992 *Clinical supervision and mentorship in nursing.* Chapman & Hall, London.

Holt, L. 1995 Clinical supervision in nursing practice. *Emergency Nurse* 3(4), 21–23.

Jarvis, P. 1992 Reflective practice and nursing. *Nurse Education Today* **12**(3), 174–181.

Jeffers, S. 1991 *Feel the fear but do it anyway.* Addison Wesley, New York.

Johns, C. 1994 Clinical notes: nuances of reflection. *Journal of Clinical Nursing* **3**, 71–75.

Kennedy, G. 1992 *The perfect negotiation – all you need to get it right first time.* Century Business, London.

Kohner, N. 1994 *Clinical supervision in practice. An executive summary.* King's Fund Centre, London.

Moss-Kanter, R. 1984 *The change masters.* Allen and Unwin, London.

Myers, I. and Briggs, K.C. 1987 *Myers–Briggs Type Indicator.* Consulting Psychologists Press, USA.

NHS Management Executive 1992 *The Patient's Charter and you.* NHSME, London.

Peters, T.J. and Waterman, R.H. 1982 *In search of excellence. Lessons from America's best run companies.* Harper Collins, London.

Plant, R. 1987 *Managing change and making it stick.* Harper Collins, London.

Proctor, B. 1991 On being a trainer. In: Dryden, W. and Thorne, B. (Eds), *Training and supervision for counselling in action.* Sage Publications, London.

Rafferty, A.M. 1991 *Leading questions.* King's Fund Centre, London.

Read, S.M., Jones, N.M.B. and Williams, B.T. 1992 Nurse Practitioners in accident and emergency departments: what do they do? *British Medical Journal* **305**, 1466–1469.

Read, S.M. and George, S. 1994 Nurse Practitioners in accident and emergency departments: reflections on a pilot study. *Journal of Advanced Nursing* **19**, 705–716.

Rees, M. and Kinnersley, P. 1996 Nurse-led management of minor illness in a GP surgery. *Nursing Times* **92**(6), 32–33.

Royal College of Nursing 1994 *Accident and emergency: challenging the boundaries.* Accident and Emergency Association.

Sbiah, L. 1994 Reaching out – nurses' role expansion. *Emergency Nurse* **1**(1), 23.

Salvage, J. 1988 Facilitating model based nursing. Unpublished paper, cited at Gateshead School of Nursing Models conference.

Schon, D. 1983 *The reflective practitioner. How professionals think in action.* Basic Books, New York.

Stewart, J. 1994 *Management of change through training and development. A change process.* Kogan Page, London.

UKCC 1990 *The report of the post-registration, education and practice project.* UKCC, London.

UKCC 1992 *The scope of professional practice.* UKCC, London.

Wallace, D. 1996 Experiential learning and critical thinking in nursing. *Nursing Standard* **10**(31), 43–47.

Walker, S. 1996 Reflective practice in the A&E setting. *Accident & Emergency Nursing* **4**(1), 27–30.

Walsh, M. 1995 Why are they so successful? *Nursing Times,* **3**(2), 4–5.

Wright, S. 1989 *Changing nursing practice* (1st edition). Edward Arnold, London.

Wright, S. 1991(a) Facilitating therapeutic nursing and independent practice. In: McMahon, R. and Pearson, A. (Eds), *Nursing as therapy*. Chapman & Hall, London.

Wright, S. 1991(b) Nursing development. *Nursing Standard* 5(38), 52–53.

Wright, S. 1996 Unlock the leadership potential. *Nursing Management* 3(2), 8–10.

CHANGING PRACTICE: CHANGING MYSELF

Sue Pearce

Participation in the Clinical Leadership course provided me with a plethora of ideas and reading options, but primarily reinforced the continual need for self-analysis and reflection as to how I approach my work.

It is easy to ask myself *who* I am and *what* I do, but to function effectively and grow with my evolving nursing role it is essential that I am more self-questioning and challenging as to my actions – *why* did I do this? and the process into achieving a target – *how* have I done this? and what have I learned?

Thinking, reflecting and learning on the job is necessary to function 'as a whole' but all too often due to pressure of time, it is the doing and moving a task along that demands all my energies and leaves little time for the former, let alone the synthesis of these combined processes.

Many have offered theories into the process of reflection, Dewey (1993) being generally acknowledged as the first to suggest that reflective thought, in the context of learning through experience, is not just problem-solving but a constant way of thinking and being.

I readily identify with Van Manen's (1977) theory which offers four levels of reflection:

1 What did I do? – reflection that is mainly descriptive.

2 How did I do it? – reflecting upon techniques required to meet objectives.

3 Have I reached my objectives / desired change?; analysing the outcome? – reflecting upon relationships between principles and practice.

4 Do I stand up for my personal beliefs or accept the situation as it is? – reflecting upon the previous levels but having concern for my own ethical, moral and political values.

The last two, more complex, options require more in-depth knowledge of self and possibly assistance from others to benefit from the reflective experience. All of the above are influenced by my personal situation at any given time, the level of my self-esteem, physical and psychological stamina, the time and support available and so on.

I have recently become acquainted with Clinical Supervision (Butterworth and Faugier, 1993) and believe his has offered me an opportunity to reflect at all of the levels Van Manen ascribes to. It is becoming more integrated into my normal daily work pattern and not an 'add on' where problems and frustrations are 'aired' over coffee or an 'if there is time later, we will talk about it' situation.

Clinical Supervision has been like finding another piece in my professional development 'jigsaw puzzle'. Using Kolb's (1984) experiential learning cycle (Fig. 6.2) it offers a framework, not only for myself, but for those whom I now supervise. By following this cycle of experience, reflection, conceptualisation and active experimentation, I can share my experience; look for solutions; develop a plan; decide if an objective is worth striving for or move on to something new. Previously, all of these concerns and difficulties would have been kept

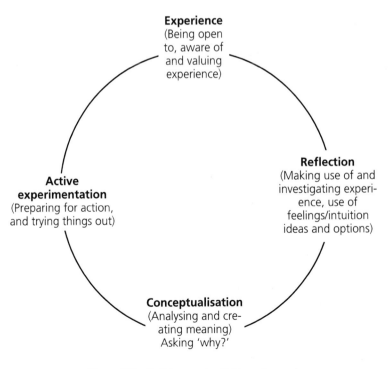

Figure 6.2 Kolb's experiential learning cycle

'locked in' or shared with someone outside the workplace, leaving some tasks or decisions 'hanging in mid-air' and blocking any learning or transition.

I will return to the impact of Clinical Supervision on my role later in this study, but will now focus on my personality type so as the reader may be more enlightened as to who I am and how this 'shapes' my clinical leadership and change management role.

McGregor (1960) offers the two options for assessing the type of human being I am, Theory X and Theory Y.

My characteristics are those fitting Theory Y – it is natural to work and be committed, so long as I am enthused and in control of tasks/objectives to be achieved. The reward for this hard work is to reach my fullest potential and get a regular boost to my ego! Accepting responsibility comes readily. It is only when the opposite is experienced that I become demotivated, frustrated and positively bored.

No doubt Theory Y characteristics are shared by most of my nursing colleagues, but I can recognise a few individuals who meet the criteria for Theory X, who McGregor describes as reluctant to work, lack enthusiasm and need directing, or even threatening, to put in adequate effort and who avoid responsibility. Perhaps these nurses are naturally Theory Y human beings but the constant pressure of the job, feeling devalued and demotivated over a long period of time has insidiously allowed Theory X characteristics to be more exposed, thus eroding their commitment and standards of patient care.

I have assessed my personality type against the Myers–Briggs Type Indicators (MBTI) (Myers and Briggs, 1987), a simplified adaptation of the theory of personality developed by Carl Jung, the psychologist. The outcome of this assessment suggests that my preferred characteristics are to be extrovert, sensing, judging and I share equally on the thinking and feeling indicators. This is reinforced by offering some common factors with each personality type.

Accordingly I can advise you that I am practical, realistic, matter of fact, like to organise and have a natural head for business! I work best with encouragement and praise and am mainly interested in the things that directly and visibly affect people's lives. All of these ring very true, and as you might have noted, are all very positive attributes.

On the more negative side I tend not to be interested in subjects that I have little use for, a prime example of this being a reluctance to learn about technical apparatus, even though it would be of benefit; I am still struggling with the complexities of the library's CD ROM even after several support sessions from the librarian. I no doubt fall into the 'IT Luddite' category!

A further characteristic suggests that I am a born cooperator but those who know me well would be quick to advise that this is not always so, and in fact can be very inflexible, questioning and downright uncooperative if I believe the situation demands it. This mode of behaviour can obviously compromise my credibility as a clinical leader and change expert if interpreted in a negative manner by those who are on the 'receiving end', but in the chaotic world I work in decisions and risks have to be taken to get the job done. Therefore, although in principle a flaw in my personality, in practice my intransigence and tenacity can be an asset when working in 'chaos' or negotiating for resources to ensure adequate staffing levels are available to meet the needs of the patients.

Nelson Mandela (1994) advises 'that when one is consistently reacting to changing circumstances, one rarely has the chance to consider carefully the ramifications of one's decisions', a statement that can surely be applied to nursing, but one which must remind me to reflect on the impact my decisions have on others. Again, the use of Clinical Supervision is now of paramount importance in assisting me to work through this process and question my behaviour and actions.

Another useful addition for self-assessment is Belbin's (1981) Team Role Self Perception Inventory. Having now completed this it offers a much clearer insight into my strengths and weaknesses as a team player.

The analysis, in general, reinforces the personal characteristics identified with McGregor's theory and MBTI. As a team member I like to complete tasks, can galvanise the team into action and help to overcome things which may go wrong, but this also suggests a streak of perfectionism and a reluctance to 'let things go'. Belbin divides leadership personality types into coordinators and shapers. My type is that of a shaper, always looking for patterns in team discussions to invite ideas and push the team towards a decision or action. I have the capacity to drive things forward, can be dynamic and challenging, but have a weakness to be impatient and allow myself to be provoked or intimidated.

I now appreciate the need to have coping strategies for dealing with the impact of stress and how, when caught off guard, I unconsciously fall into the 'victim role', feeling useless and isolated. As Maya Angelou (1993) advises 'Whining is not only graceless, but can be dangerous. It can alert a brute that a victim is in the neighbourhood'.

It is true, but I must be aware of not allowing myself to turn into 'the brute' when faced with challenging individuals or situations. Becoming more self-aware and participating in group supervision has reassured me that this tendency is one I share with many others and certainly with the majority of nurses!

Why is this trait of falling into 'victim role' so common? Perhaps it is the nature of our nursing role, the historical need to ensure that everything is done properly, with no allowances for mistakes, however minor. Salvage (1985) suggests that exposure to senior nurses behaving in a heartless and insulting way creates individuals who are insecure, lack confidence and evolve to behave in a similar way as a form of self-protection. Even with a more open supportive management approach it would appear that wearing down this collective 'mind set' in nursing is a long evolving process but one which I strive to achieve for myself and others.

The perfectionist in me also influences the sometimes unrealistic expectations I set myself, thus when I do not achieve them, my initial instinct is to feel a failure and again fall into the victim role. I am slowly learning to temper my objectives and develop a more structured approach to my work – the work better, not harder principle.

This being said, the need for credible support systems in nursing is essential. Rafferty (1991) states 'It is of vital importance to provide good support and supervision systems for leaders. A structure for development and challenge is critical'.

At the other end of the nursing spectrum, students are now offered preceptorship and mentorship through their training and whilst establishing themselves in clinical practice. Butterworth and Faugier (1993) offer a definition of the terms 'mentor and perceptor' as a prelude to debating and clarifying the need to establish Clinical Supervision in all areas of nursing. They advise that supervision cannot be imposed arbitrarily on nurses, but it surely must be the best option available for creating the support and supervision systems that nurses, at all levels, require to assist learning through reflection.

Tschudin and Schober (1990) suggest that the basis of self-management is to listen to yourself, others and the environment, therefore are able to hear what is happening and will be more equipped to bring about change.

Bearing all of these analyses and theories in mind I believe that I am honest, sincere, conscientious, hardworking and committed. I have a well organised pragmatic approach to my work and can be very determined and passionate when championing the way forward for the patients, staff and services I am accountable for.

The scope for self-assessment is endless and I have chosen to reveal characteristics and opinions that I feel comfortable sharing with the reader. To delve too deeply and explore too much of myself is beyond the scope of this study.

My nursing credentials are firmly entrenched in District Nursing, working for 16 years as a District Nursing Sister until 1992 when I achieved the post of Professional Adviser (H grade). This new role came about as part of an exercise to reduce nurse management, the main core of the job being to offer operational support to a General Clinical Manager and District Nursing staff in a given locality and carry a half-time caseload.

The reality of the role is far more demanding than the written job description portrays, but it has certainly challenged, stretched and at times, overwhelmed me. As the District Nursing Service has been impacted upon by more highly dependent patients, early and often inappropriate discharges from hospital, GP fundholding, Patient's Charter bandings and Post-Registration Education and Practice (PREP) requirements to name but a few, all at a time when resources in community care are wanting as the needs of individuals referred are more complex.

At the present time I am Acting Clinical Manager and have responsibility for District Nurses working in Primary Health Care Teams. This role is challenging and is developing my clinical leadership, change agency and management skills, knowledge base, decision-making skills and assertiveness. As I took on the role during a major restructuring within the Community Directorate, it has certainly tested my capabilities to cope at this level.

Rafferty (1993) describes this as circumstantial leadership in that it is a role determined by expectations of the group or organisation – effective leaders adapt their style to the demands of the situation.

In a description of 'Coping Management' (Marsh and MacAlpine, 1995), I am aware that my focus is on the immediate work to be done within the given resources which are available to me. I have certainly developed competencies in the 'fire fighting' and 'papering over the cracks' approaches to management. This being so I hopefully ensure that all essential care for patients is carried out, staff supported in their work and the budget is as balanced as it can be!

There is little time for team meetings with staff, service development, analysis of needs for patients, staff and myself, but my time out for Clinical Supervision has been essential in assisting me through this transition. It is certainly creating a much firmer base from which I work.

This opportunity is allowing me to assume clinical leadership at different levels and I now question how credible I can be to provide this at present, when distanced from 'bedside' nursing. During the past few months I have provided no direct patient care as the job demands a more administrative, indirect influence on care provision and operational issues.

Ashton (1996) offers some comparison between one who leads and one who manages, and even though some shared competencies and assets are offered, he suggests that the manager role deals with the resourcing and smooth running of the system and ensuring the job gets done, whereas the leader role concentrates on the potential of the staff and organisation – having a vision, communicating and sharing with others. Motivating and pulling the threads of ideas together to drive the way forward turning the vision into reality.

Another overview is provided by Rafferty (1991) who discusses the visible and less visible approaches to clinical leadership. Her findings suggest one leadership style as being visible and charismatic or high profile and the other less visible, facilitative and ordinary. My present role influences a more visible style, presenting positive images to and for the District Nursing Service, being more dynamic in a wider field with other professionals and hanging onto my values and principles when under pressure.

When in my Professional Adviser role, all the above apply but in a less visible way, impacting more informally on the staff and direct patient care, offering a more insidious but incremental approach to my clinical leadership role.

Rafferty goes on to debate the constraints on potential clinical leaders and offers some analysis on what is holding nurses back from developing this role.

Language, values and culture systems were identified as being different from the new general management 'settlers' who have now colonised the NHS. Rafferty's interviewees advised that the task of leadership in nursing was to rescue the profession from being seen as an invisible but necessary service. I suggest that much needs to be done on a national and at a local level but the nursing profession must look to its own 'internal' language, values and cultures to ensure we are all aiming for the same goals and sharing the same vision. Territorialism and tribal systems still exist and are actively flourishing in nursing, acting as barriers to better communication, understanding of roles and effective teamwork.

In District Nursing this occurs because teams work in relative isolation from their colleagues and distanced from central management. This picture is now more complicated by GP fundholding and the confusion of loyalties experienced by District Nurses – 'which tribe do I belong to? the District Nurse tribe or the GP tribe?' Learning the language, values and culture of contracting with fundholders will also be an enormous achievement for any nurse who succeeds!

Fortunately, moves are afoot locally where a pilot scheme is currently in process with an aim to encourage primary health care nurses to work more effectively together. It offers a strategy to harness the skills of District Nurses, Health Visitors and Practice Nurses involved, encouraging better communication and a framework in which to address the nursing needs of their practice population. Hopefully, this will not only break down territorial and tribal barriers but will result in stronger expert teams, where potential clinical leaders can be nurtured and developed.

Recently I have read Nelson Mandela's autobiography and many times he refers to the traditional leadership and tribal systems and the difficulties it created during his struggle against apartheid. I find this thought-provoking and it reinforces my belief that nurses must stop the 'infighting' and be aware of the image portrayed to those outside

the profession, before they can be credited as having strong professional leaders.

Rafferty advises that investment into nursing research is wanting
and the internal market is potentially depressing future investment.
Who will invest locally and nationally if visible, high profile nurse
leaders and managers do not present a shared vision based on clinical
knowledge and mutual respect?

But on a more positive note some individuals and nursing groups
are achieving this and influencing improved patient care, often in a
multi-agency setting. Nursing Development Units are becoming more
common place and individual practitioners having real impact on their
specialist area of work.

Webber (1993) is one such example. Her paper on the changing role
of the Macmillan Nurse is influencing the way forward in this area and
demonstrating the need for an evolving approach to nursing care to
meet the changing needs of those we care for. The framework Webber
offers for the evolving role of the Macmillan Nurse is proving very
useful in redefining my Professional Adviser role and assisting in
rewriting the job description. I believe this exercise will provide clarity
and a more patient-centred/staff support approach rather than
responsibilities generated from organisational changes.

Wille (1992) states that leaders are there to help people do a better
job. They are responsible for putting the system right when necessary.
The better the system becomes the more chance workers have of doing
a good job.

In my role I need to balance my time between direct and indirect
care and work in a more structured system offering clinical research-
based practice, clinical leadership and operational support, as well as
promoting and developing Clinical Supervision and providing line
management support as delegated.

One such service I lead is the Community Nursing Bathing Service.
Assisting in the development, launching, maintaining and line managing this new service has been a very exciting opportunity for me. It
focuses on my clinical leadership and change management roles and
how they impact upon this staff group, service provision and future
development, demonstrating the how and why of my reflective practice.

Before commencing the pilot scheme for this service it was essential
to gain the support of the District Nursing Sisters to ensure a sound
understanding of the admission criteria and their future role in the
assessment process. It would also mean a degree of 'letting go' of what
had traditionally been a component of the District Nurse's caseload.

Upon reflection I now appreciate that my skills as a change agent
were somewhat lacking, but Turrell (1996) cites an Equation for
Individual Change Education (Fig. 6.3). This now provides me with a

If an individual is willing to change s/he will only engage if:

A + B + C > (lessens) the pain of change

A = Dissatisfaction of the current situation

B = Anticipation of a better future

C = A practical first step

Figure 6.3 Individual change equation. After Turrell (1996)

focus when planning change, but at the time of the service launch my objective was very 'woolly' and I naively thought that my vision and enthusiasm would be shared by my colleagues.

Wright (1996a) advises that change is never linear and can be messy and unpredictable. I certainly learned the hard way and even though a direct informative style of leadership can get a project up and running, it needs to be balanced with listening to, encouraging and empowering staff to offer and debate alternatives for service provision. Hansell and Salter (1995) support this view and reinforce previous discussion regarding the listening to others more, instead of telling them what to do. If this style is never modified, motivation will decline and nothing will get done when the leader is not there.

I don't believe my behaviour at that time was over-authoritarian; my personal vision was very clear in my mind, but it took much longer for others to accept at a time of many changes. Now over two years later, the service is well accepted and integrated to the care planning menu on offer.

The change has been incremental as the service was gradually introduced Borough-wide. The news soon spread that this was a high quality service of real benefit. The courteous, competent care being provided by the Bathing Attendants and the commitment of the Co-ordinator was evident. This was very reassuring and provided evidence that my time-consuming role as a 'gatekeeper' was paying off.

For me this included looking for certain competencies and personal characteristics in an individual, at the time of interview, with the objective of employing those who provided evidence of a high standard of patient-focused care, advocated for the patients and ensured a good image for the service.

Generally that has been very successful, and apart from the isolated negative incident, I now have a team who more than meet the essential criteria required.

Having this responsibility has been an excellent learning opportunity in that I have developed skills and knowledge in selection and recruitment, am more aware of Equal Opportunities and employment legislation, but also understand the importance of 'gatekeeping' to strive for the best possible qualities in staff in the desire to provide a quality service.

Interestingly it has also offered an opportunity to develop these competencies for some District Nursing Sisters and now the interview panel will comprise of at least one Sister, the lead interviewer role is often rotated and the planning of the interview questions is a shared team effort. This offers an example of my leadership role as servant, as described by Wright (1996b). He uses the analysis of a flock of snowgeese in flight to describe how the leader falls back after creating the air turbulence, and allows another to take over the lead for a time. This style is one I now appreciate and provides me with a sense of satisfaction as others start to take more responsibility and the associated risks, gain more confidence and ownership of their work.

As cited earlier, Rafferty (1991) advises that nurses must respond and seize the research agenda. I am pleased to advise the reader that the Bathing Service is 'pure nurse' researched, developed, maintained and marketed, but the direct patient care is provided by 'unqualified' nursing assistants, and on a day-to-day basis led by two very competent, but unqualified, coordinators.

Perhaps to the staff of this service I am seen as a 'clinical expert'. Wright (1996b) terms this leader as a 'connoisseur' of nursing and the system. I am the one who may know what to do and act as a resource for clinical or organisational information. But over time the staff are now less likely to contact me in the first instance, but consult with the coordinators who have now a firmer knowledge base and increasing expertise. Ashton (1996) describes this as a general supervision role where subordinates have the freedom to exercise discretion in their work rather than having tight controls over them.

A further trait is to have the ability to rise above a situation and assess it objectively, taking all the facts into account, prioritising actions before descending and dealing with it. This is often termed the 'helicopter trait'.

I am aware that my leadership is imposed on the Bathing Service Team, just as in all areas of nursing (and the wider world). Few of us are in a position to choose who leads us; this responsibility is acquired by successful selection or being delegated the leadership tasks.

Bernhard and Walsh (1981) suggest that imposed leadership can affect team functioning and accord. The leader may have a more difficult time being accepted and gaining team support.

Comparisons are made with the emergent leader; one who has 'natural' leadership style and tends to automatically take on the role, or one who incrementally acquires the skills, confidence and trust of others to acquire the lead. In this instance my imposed leadership has not created difficulties and the two coordinators have emerged as 'natural' leaders.

Facilitating the training and development of this staff group is another element of my role. Encouraging debate within the team as to skills and knowledge they require assists planning of training sessions but also appraising and building on existing competencies is essential. Egan (1986) offers a positive management approach to helping, more often used in the therapeutic setting, but provides a framework to assist staff grow and want to learn more. Egan suggests that 'Clients are our customers and have a right to expect the best service from us'. Nurturing this philosophy assists in creating a focus for learning while it offers a positive experience and a rationale for staff to 'own' their own learning and remain eager to take up any learning opportunity offered.

This approach appears to be working and training sessions and meetings are a time for sharing and mutual support which often act as 'informal supervision' sessions.

It is interesting to compare this staff group's willingness and uninhibited manner of sharing feelings and problems with that of a group of experienced and trained nurses who tend to be economic with their real feelings and focus on factual operational problems. This is perhaps evidence that this new breed of nursing assistant is being nurtured and supported in a more 'staff friendly' environment where respect is shown for how people feel as well as how they perform – investing in people in its truest sense.

Maintaining this approach and responding to staff needs promotes a safe, caring environment, and basing these needs on Maslow's (1978) hierarchy can raise self-esteem in individuals and create an environment where job satisfaction and self-fulfilment are the norm.

Using this assignment as a 'vehicle' for reflection, self-analysis, evidence of competencies and an insight into what I do, I will now bring this 'journey' to a close and can confirm Henry Kissinger's statement that 'Leadership is not always quite what you would expect it to be!'.

How do I measure as a clinical leader and change agent? I feel comfortable in the role, ordinary and not overwhelmed by its many visible and less visible elements. I cannot assume that I have the right to bestow the title upon myself but will leave it to those I support and impact upon to decide if I have earned it!

References

Angelou, M. 1993 *Wouldn't take nothing for my journey now.* Virago, London.

Ashton, F. 1996 *Discussion paper, Clinical Leadership course.* Clearwater Consultancy, Mossley.

Belbin, R.M. 1981 *Mangement teams.* Heinemann, Oxford.

Bernard, W. 1981 *Leadership.* McGraw-Hill, New York.

Butterworth, T. and Faugier, J. 1993 *Clinical supervision.* Heinemann, London.

Dewey, D. 1993 *How we think.* D C Heath, Boston, MA.

Egan, G. 1986 *The skilled helper* (3rd Edition). Books/Cole, Monterey, CA.

Hansell, D. and Salter, S. 1995 *The clinician's management handbook.* W B Saunders, London.

Kolb, D.A. (1984) *Experiential learning experience as the source of learning and development.* Prentice Hall, Eaglewood, NJ.

Mandela, N. 1994 *Long walk to freedom.* Abacus, London.

Marsh, S. and MacAlpine, M. 1995 *Our own capabilities.* King's Fund, London.

Maslow, A. 1970 *Motivation and personality* (2nd Edition). Harper and Row, New York.

McGregor, D. 1960 *The human side of enterprise.* McGraw-Hill, New York.

Myers, I. and Briggs, K.C. 1987 *Myers–Briggs Type Indicator.* Consulting Psychologists Press Inc., USA.

Rafferty, A.M. 1993 *Leading questions.* King's Fund, London.

Salvage, J. 1985 *The politics of nursing.* Heinemann, London.

Tschudin, V. and Schober, J. 1990 *Managing yourself: essentials of nurse management.* Macmillan, London.

Turrell, A. 1966 NHS management cuts. Unpublished paper. Queen's University Hospital, Nottingham.

Van Manen, M. 1977 Linking ways of knowing with way of being practical. *Curriculum Inquiry* **1**(7), 14.

Webber, J. 1993 *The evolving role of the Macmillan Nurse: discussion paper.* Cancer Relief Macmillan Fund, London.

Wille, E. 1992 *Quality: achieving excellence.* Century, London.

Wright, S. 1996(a) The need to develop nursing practice through innovation and practice change. *International Journal of Clinical Nursing* **2**, 142–148.

Wright, S. 1996(b) Unlock the leadership potential. *Nursing Management* **3**(2), 8–10.

MACMILLAN RESPITE AT HOME SCHEME – MY ROLE IN CHANGE

Helena Kearsley

Introduction

The topic of this section relates to the 'Macmillan Respite at Home Scheme', which was a new service launched in June 1996. I am the key facilitator for the service and aim here to demonstrate my leadership role and change agency skills.

My present role

Before I proceed further, I think it is important to introduce my present role and where I am at. I am the Professional Adviser for District Nursing for Stockport Healthcare NHS Trust. This is split into:

1 Half-time clinical post which involves managing a small caseload of two single-handed GPs.

2 Half-time Professional Adviser role i.e. resource for any clinical issues appertaining to District Nursing to all District Nursing Teams within Stockport Healthcare Trust:
   - revising/developing District Nursing protocols,
   - supporting/advising staff with operational issues,
   - active participation of recruitment/selection of District Nursing staff within the Trust.

I was requested by the Clinical Director of the Primary and Public Health Directorate to undertake and facilitate this scheme from as far back as June 1995, as originally this scheme was to be launched in September 1995; but funding was withdrawn and a fresh bid reapplied. Funding for the scheme comes two-thirds from the Cancer Relief Macmillan Fund and one-third from Stockport Health Authority.

What is the scheme?

- It is a free service to all Stockport residents over 16 years of age who have cancer or a terminal illness.
- It is a service to enable people to be cared for at home during their final year of life.
- It will operate as a pilot scheme to a budget of £40 000 for 18 months.
- Stockport is one of the seven sites to participate in these pilot schemes funded by Cancer Relief Macmillan Fund.
- The remaining six sites are Pontefract, Carlisle, Solihull, Kettering, Norwich and Aylesbury.
- The need for this service was identified by the Review of Palliative Care Services undertaken by Stockport Health Authority in October 1994, which highlighted deficits in service provision, often resulting in patients being admitted to hospital when it was not their desire to be there.

Aims of the scheme

- To provide intensive direct and indirect care, but usually short-term support to patients suffering from cancer or other terminal illnesses.
- This will be a supplementary service to the existing main services provided, such as the District Nursing Service and any Social Services input.

Objectives of the scheme

- To offer crisis intervention when normal support mechanisms have failed e.g. if the main carer is ill or needs a break.
- To provide support for patients following major surgery or chemotherapy / radiotherapy i.e. may be an individual with young children, the latter need collecting from school and meals made for them and staying with them until partner returns home from work.
- To provide support for patients, which will enable those whose wish it is, to be cared for at home.
- To provide support which will reduce incidence of hospital admissions unless it is the desired option.

What is my role in this scheme?

I am the key facilitator for the scheme i.e. the operational side of the service. For this function to be fulfilled, I have to demonstrate my role in implementation of the service and my leadership skills in changing the delivery of the service.

I based my style around Hersey and Blanchard's (1976) situational leadership: 'Leadership seems to be something to do with knowing what the requirements of the task (or objectives) to be achieved are and getting things done through people'.

In 'Leading Questions' (Rafferty, 1993) a working definition to be considered might be 'Leadership is the ability to identify a goal, come up with a strategy for achieving that goal and inspire your team to join you in putting that strategy into action'.

Invariably people (staff) present as many problems/challenges to the leader as the objectives and tasks of the job itself (Hersey and Blanchard, 1976). This brings me back to my role within the scheme and the first part of that was implementation of the scheme. I knew what the requirements of the task were and I needed a strategy to achieve them.

As mentioned earlier, this scheme was launched in June 1996. In view of that, a large amount of the preparatory work had commenced and been achieved. One of the earliest tasks I had to undertake was the preparation of the documentation for the service:

- referral forms
- assessment forms
- service information leaflets for patients and carers
- flyers to introduce the service to District Nurses, Health Visitors, Social Workers and GPs.

As this scheme was funded by Cancer Relief Macmillan Fund, a named Macmillan Nurse had to be included in the facilitation of the scheme. Together we designed, altered and redesigned numerous times the above documentation, which was finally approved, printed and ready for the launch.

The next item on the agenda was to set up a meeting with the Departmental Head of Statistics to organise statistical data collection.

Recruitment and selection were next – the first advertisement drew a very poor response and judging by the applications, the calibre of the candidates was inappropriate. A second advertisement, totally reworded, attracted 25 applicants. I was looking to run the scheme with either five part-time staff or two full-time and one part-time. Five part-time staff were preferred as this gave greater flexibility, but from the applications, literally all applicants were looking for full-time jobs.

The interview panel consisted of myself, the Macmillan Nurse and the Acting Clinical Manager who shortlisted the applicants to 12. We successfully recruited two full-time and one part-time B grade personnel who commenced on 10 June 1996.

I learnt a valuable lesson from the recruitment process – I was not entirely satisfied with the wording of the first advertisement which had been drafted by a previous manager. I should have used my skills of diplomacy and negotiation to 'persuade' the Clinical Director to my viewpoint – i.e. the wording for the first advertisement was not right and should have been rewritten, which we did later. Readvertisements, which in this case achieved our goal, cost time and money.

Planning the induction and the level/amount of training for the new team came next. The Macmillan Nurse and I consulted with the Training Manager for the Trust.

Apart from the core induction for all new employees, the training had to include topics such as bereavement, grief and coping with difficult questions. The Macmillan Trust had been delegated to undertake these particular topics. I selected three District Nursing Sisters to help with the orientation of the new team – each member spent some time working with the District Nursing Sister to understand the input of the District Nursing Service.

As these staff could be involved in food preparation, arrangements were made for them to attend a Food Hygiene course, as well as the mandatory Moving and Handling training session.

A 'Welcome' first day package with provision of lunch by a nutrition representative was organised to:

- welcome the team as a group
- introduce all involved within the scheme
- outline the aims of the scheme
- outline expectations of the scheme and of the team
- outline what the team could expect from their leaders
- recognise stress/stressors.

I believe the 'first day package' was important to the team and towards the success of the scheme.

One asks 'what is a team?'

- A team is an effective working group.
- Our social needs and our self-esteem needs can be satisfied through membership of an effective group.
- Team development is a process of removing obstacles that prevent the team functioning effectively and planning how to improve the team's overall performance.

I believe in the theory of 'leader as a servant' (Wright, 1996) – working as a change agent to help others develop and put into practice their own vision of ideals, building relationships and facilitating their own growth.

I want the team to feel valued and nurtured and for its members to have peer support with each other, apart from what their leaders can give. The scheme's success will be achieved through the team's motivation and commitment. O'Connor (1968) lists some of the general reasons for motivation:

- genuine interest
- a wish to perform the task well
- conforming to standards
- looking for recognition from colleagues
- in order to please
- in order not to disappoint
- a better salary if success is achieved. If success is achieved, it will mean continuation of the scheme, meaning that their employment continues.

I have no doubts that the team, being employed for a new service, possesses these reasons to be, and feel, motivated.

The selected team has a genuine interest in this particular field of work and because its members are aware it is a pilot scheme, they wish to seek recognition from their colleagues. As mentioned earlier, even though I do not doubt the team's motivation, I am also very aware that due to the nature and intensity of the work the scheme offers, the team is very vulnerable to stress. The members need to be able to recognise their own signals and I need to exercise my 'listening' skills.

Selye (1976) says that 'Stress is a non-specific response of the body to any demand, whether it is caused by, or results in, pleasant or unpleasant conditions'.

Stress is non-specific; everyone reacts differently and has different signs, which is why it is so difficult to pin down and people who are experiencing it are so often not believed. McNeel (1987) states 'If people say they are stressed or exhibit stress symptoms, they should be believed. What feels real has a basis in reality'.

Whilst stress is a necessary factor for survival, when it leads to an excessive demand on an individual and beyond his/her ability to cope, stress becomes destructive. The result of too much stress is a person's total inability to function effectively.

As the team leader, I need to to be very aware of these signals and to be able to offer support when needed. I schedule monthly meetings with the team with two main goals:

1 For the team to meet together, reinforcing peer support and build up rapport, relationship, and build confidence to be proactive and take responsibility.
2 For the team members to be able to discuss their concerns, worries or simply just to 'air' feelings. Any areas of conflict are hopefully constructively managed.

Whilst these meetings are structured with an agenda, there is allocated time for each team member to have his/her say. I am also available for any individual personal consultation.

Having recruited the staff and being aware that the staff can present as many problems/challenges to the leader as the objectives and tasks of the job itself, the next step of implementation was to launch the scheme.

The District Nurses became the main assessors of the scheme – i.e. they were requested to assess the patient and environment prior to the input of the scheme, unless the patient was already known to the referring District Nursing Sister. This could have been viewed by some as 'extra work' and could have caused resentment/resistance. For this reason I feel it was very important that the launch and marketing of the scheme was at the right pitch.

The Macmillan Nurse and I decided that we would launch the scheme initially to the District Nurses only, as they were the main users of the scheme. We selected four locality areas of Stockport and dates for these 'roadshows' were distributed to District Nurses in all clinics. The Macmillan Nurse and I selected an area each and the remaining two areas were delegated to the Acting Clinical Manager and Manager for Public Health Nursing (both of whom are of District Nursing background and had been involved in the planning network of the scheme).

This scheme comes under the remit of the responsibilities of the Public Health Clinical Manager. I wanted the launch/marketing of the scheme to have a personal touch, rather than just distributing flyers and service information leaflets in the post.

Attendance at the 'roadshows' by the District Nurses was very impressive. There was a lot of interest and enthusiasm and the majority felt it was the 'booster' which had been needed for a long time.

Some of the negativity expressed surrounded the issue of the limited resources of the scheme (which would probably mean operating a waiting list) and the maximum limit of the service to any one client for a period of seven days. These issues were discussed and explanations given for the criteria. The three of us who were involved in the launch of the scheme were able to reassure the groups that although criteria for any service have to be established, nothing is written in 'tablets of stone'.

If, for instance, on the seventh day that a patient is in receipt of the scheme, the patient concerned is extremely ill e.g. 'Cheyne-Stoking' and is close to death, then I or the Macmillan Nurse will make the decision to reassess that situation and possibly extend the length of service. However, that ultimate decision-making process rests with me or the Macmillan Nurse. This will absolve the District Nurses from that onerous task and will not compromise their relationship with their patients and carers.

At the launch, the majority of the District Nurses were convinced of the benefits such a scheme would bring to enhance their own existing

District Nursing Services. The scheme was introduced to other health-care professionals soon after it became operational. These included the Hospital Liaison staff, GPs, Health Visitors and Social Workers.

That covers the main aspects of the implementation process. The 'smaller tasks' associated with it were:

- Selecting and purchasing a 'uniform' for the staff – the colour for Macmillan is green, so it was decided to supply green polo shirts/trousers/skirts/sweatshirts with the Healthcare logo.
- Purchasing of mobile telephones for the three team members and myself (Macmillan Nurse will cover when I am off). This was felt to be essential, as it needs to be a fast, responsive service, and I need to be able to access the staff. Whilst waiting for referrals or if not utilised on the scheme, the staff will be used to help the District Nursing Teams who have understood that the member of the scheme may have to return their list of patients to the District Nursing team at short notice.

The new staff began work on 10 June 1996 for their induction and training. At this point, reflecting on the change and leadership skills/style I have used, I found myself using a more active/participative one from 10 June 1996. I have found it necessary to endeavour to be flexible in the way I deal with people, for example, some respond well to a supportive style, some need a more prescriptive style.

Much depends on:

- the willingness/unwillingness of the individual or group
- the ability/inability of the individual or group
- maturity is another important factor to consider.

Simple framework to explain

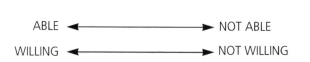

Willingness is to do with motivation/attitude. Everyone fits some-where along each scale – take the simplest approach to intersect the two scales. Ability is to do with skill/knowledge.

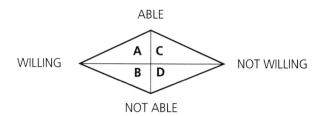

A   People who are both willing and able can usually work with little supervision but will always still need support. These staff will generally be experienced / mature / motivated.

B   People who are willing but not able need both support and direction (prescriptive leadership). May apply to new staff needing training and experience.

C   People who are able but not willing could need both supportive and prescriptive leadership e.g. when confronted with change may adopt 'I prefer to do it my way – I've always worked this way, it's the way we do things here'.

D   When people start work it is generally thought that whilst they may not be able to do the job totally effectively, they at least have a willingness to learn – as in B above.

It would be good to have everyone in category A or B. However, staff with experience sometimes display dissatisfaction / demotivation / relationship difficulties which take them into C. Supportive leadership hopefully helps them to resolve their difficulties by counselling.

If this fails, however, a more prescriptive approach may be necessary and the leader may well say 'I hear what you say, we've tried it your way but it's not working well enough – now I want us to take a fresh approach because things need to change' (Hersey and Blanchard, 1976).

I would like to think that the recruited staff fall mainly into category A and perhaps borderline B. They are very willing and able people with experience, but need adaptation of their past experience into the new job, which I truly believe will be covered by the induction and training, plus on-going support from myself and the Macmillan Nurse. Together we aim to deliver this service to the residents of Stockport.

Outcomes

The outcomes were twofold:

1   *Initial*
- for the recruited staff to receive the necessary induction / training
- for the project to be launched on time
- for the service to be well received
- for the Stockport residents to benefit from the service.

2   *Final*
- for the scheme to be successful so that it will continue after its 18 months pilot.

Evaluation

It was decided to engage the services of Professor David Clark and his team from the University of Sheffield and Trent Palliative Care Centre to undertake the evaluation process during the pilot.

This is an area that has caused us some worry and concern from a sensitivity issue e.g. after what time interval does one send a 'patient satisfaction questionnaire' to the bereaved relatives? It is one of those situations where it is never at a right time. If it is left for too long after death, it may be resurrecting painful memories. Professor Clark and his team are also undertaking the evaluation for the other six pilot sites. He and his team will make contact with the relatives requesting permission to participate in the process and the questionnaires will be sent direct to the relatives/carers.

I will relate patient details i.e. name, address, date of birth, etc. to the team at set intervals, and inform them when death has occurred.

The results of the evaluation will only be known after the pilot study is completed in 1998.

Conclusion – self-reflection

The most important lesson I have learnt in launching the project is the amount of time preparatory work for the launch incurs. That was probably the most difficult part of the scheme.

'This is where understanding of many features (e.g. the task in hand; the needs of the group; staff empowerment, support and motivation; effective delegation; involvement of all members) is so important. Most crucial of all is to be a leader of vision with a strong sense of commitment, able to inspire others to share that vision. For the sake of the leader's sanity, it is also essential to be a "centred human being" with "head and heart"' (Wright, 1996). I can relate to this because in the stages where some of the difficulties seemed 'unsolvable' I was able to continue my 'vision', as I believe in and understand my own strength and limits, and know that being in harmony with myself is essential to creating harmony outside.

When I began this project, my MBTI (see Donna Davenport's earlier study in this chapter, p. 108) indicator was ISTJ – authoritarian and direct; respecting hierarchy. It also indicated someone responsible and earning success by concentration and thoroughness. I like to think that rather than being authoritarian, I have adopted a democratic/flexible approach. I would not have been able to achieve the preparation required for this scheme without being responsive to changes/needs, flexibility, and open-endedness, and being direct and honest.

I feel positive that towards the completion of this project, I am re-evaluating my own values, which ultimately will have an impact on my values and those of other colleagues, will help me to explore and exercise skills in democratic leadership and will heighten my skills in negotiation as that is very much needed in introducing change in practice. For this scheme to be successful, I have to help facilitate change in practice for it to be accepted. Although Adair (1989) maintains the path to leadership is open to all, this is somewhat contradicted by the fact that not everyone wishes to lead, or has the ability or confidence to do so. I believe that I have greatly enhanced these two skills.

Listing some of the skills employed to undertake this project:

- organising meetings efficiently
- leading meetings effectively
- understanding the task
- understanding the needs of the group
- understanding individual needs
- empowerment
- involvement of all members
- support and motivation
- developing relationships with others in the group
- coordinating the workload efficiently
- introducing change in practice.

References

Adair, J. 1989 *Great leaders*. Pan Books, London.

Briggs, K.C. and Myers, I. 1980 *Gifts differing*. Consulting Psychologists Press Inc., Palo Alto, CA.

Hersey, P. and Blanchard, K.H. 1976 *Situational leadership*. University Associates, Mansfield.

McNeel, B.T. 1987 *Stress*. SPCK, London.

O'Connor, K. 1968 *Learning: an introduction*. Macmillan, London.

Rafferty, A.M. 1993 *Leading questions*. King's Fund Centre, London.

Selye, H. 1976 *The stress of life* (2nd Edition). McGraw-Hill, London.

Wright, S.G. 1996 Unlock the leadership potential. *Nursing Management* **3** (2), 8–10.

7 Costs and conflicts

Lesley Surman with Stephen Wright

Stresses and strains on the staff
Clinical supervision – the essential principles
Clinical supervision – the common models
Stress and support
Staff changes
The client's perceptions
Change is a personal journey
Change agents may become laggards too!
'Tall poppy' syndrome
Financial implications

(Wilde was to be charged a large fee for an operation.) 'Ah, well then,' said Oscar, 'I suppose that I shall have to die beyond my means.'

R. H. Sherard, *Life of Oscar Wilde*

Resources required to meet change cover a wide area, but one which immediately comes to mind is that of finance, probably because it always seems to be the greatest battle and loudest niggle within the service. However, other aspects need to be considered such as the effects on the personnel involved, including the change agent and all the others affected by the change process.

Stresses and strains on the staff

The cost to individuals can be far-reaching, and is identifiable in both positive and negative terms. Innovators are, by nature of their pursuit, faced with many stresses; the first being how to approach the challenge of change to achieve success, and yet minimise the personal conflicts. Thomson (1977) identifies that over-anxiety resulting in annoyance or anger can undermine objectivity and concentration. He also suggests that 'indifference, half-heartedness, over-confidence, are equally disturbing: persistence and appreciation can only come from a certain degree of interest and concern. A moderate but effective motivation is needed'. Each individual will have to appraise themselves to identify and recognise the point at which they need to switch off (even if it be for a short period) and perhaps withdraw from the situation in order to maintain their physical, psychological and emotional well-being.

Stress can manifest itself in many ways. The change agent must recognise signs and symptoms of stress in themselves and adopt strategies to overcome these in order that he/she doesn't reach burnout, and also the change agent must recognise signs of stress in the target group and intervene when and where appropriate.

Cooper *et al.* (1988) have identified the major symptoms of stress and these can be summarised under three main headings.

Each individual appraises the stressfulness of a situation uniquely; the view, opinions, emotions and circumstances all have a bearing on the way we think and feel about ourselves. Bailey (1985) summarises that stress results from:

- The way we think about ourselves and our circumstances.
- The meaning we give to the demands we consider are being made on us.
- The value we put on the importance of caring for others.

The psychologist Chernis (1980) has suggested that burnout is a type of disease as a result of overcommitment, and later suggested that burnout meant the 'withdrawal from work in response to excessive stress or dissatisfaction'. Lazarus and Lannier (1981) define coping as 'an individual's attempt to manage (to master, tolerate, reduce, minimise, etc.) internal and external environmental demands or conflicts which tax one's resources'.

One of the first attempts at coping with stress is recognising that it exists. Change agents in leadership positions need to have sufficient awareness to recognise it in themselves, but, when they do not, this is the point where the supportive managers or colleagues should step in. The change agent needs also to be able to recognise stress effects on others. Stress which produces the kind of negative effects (as opposed to the positive ones of stimulation and motivation at work) as listed above is a sign that things are going wrong.

- Does the change agent lack the skills or knowledge to do the job?
- Are they expecting too much of themselves too quickly?
- Are the resources inadequate to meet the change requirements?
- Are the support methods failing (e.g. has the support from managers or colleagues dissipated)?

Table 7.1 Major symptoms of stress (after Cooper et al., 1988)

Physical symptoms of stress	Mental symptoms of stress	Stress-related ailments
Lack of appetite	Constant irritability with people	Hypertension: high blood pressure
Craving for food when under pressure	Feeling unable to cope	Coronary thrombosis: heart attack
Frequent indigestion or heartburn	Lack of interest in life	Migraine
Constipation or diarrhoea	Constant or recurrent fear of disease	Hay fever and allergies
Insomnia	A feeling of being a failure	Asthma
Constant tiredness	A feeling of being bad or of self-hatred	Pruritus: intense itching
Tendency to sweat for no good reason	Difficulty in making decisions	Peptic ulcers
Nervous twitches	A feeling of ugliness	Constipation
Nail-biting	Loss of interest in other people	Colitis
Headaches	Awareness of suppressed anger	Menstrual difficulties
Cramps and muscle spasms	Inability to show true feelings	Nervous dyspepsia: flatulence and indigestion
Nausea	A feeling of being the target of other people's animosity	Overactive thyroid gland
Breathlessness without exertion	Loss of sense of humour	Diabetes mellitus
Fainting spells	Feeling of neglect	Skin disorders
Frequent crying or desire to cry	Dread of the future	Tuberculosis
Impotence or frigidity	A feeling of having failed as a person or parent	Depression
Inability to sit still without fidgeting	A feeling of having no confidence	
High blood pressure	Difficulty in concentrating	
	The inability to finish one task before rushing on to the next	
	An intense fear of open or enclosed spaces or of being alone	

It may mean that stress on the change agents and their colleagues can put the whole change process into question. There has been a tendency in nursing to find a scapegoat when things go wrong. It is too easy to focus, for example, on the change agent. Salvage (1988) notes that when nurses complain that they cannot cope, the nurse is often held to blame, instead of examining the situation which has produced the failure to cope.

A full discussion on the subject of stress is beyond the scope of this text, but it needs to be recognised that stress is an inevitable part of the change process. Stress may produce either positive or negative effects on the staff, depending upon its degree of intensity. What is stressful to one person, producing a negative reaction, is simply stimulating to another. The stress usually arises not because of any failings in the change agents or their colleagues, rather as a result of problems with the planning or carrying through of the change process. Some points to consider to alleviate the situation include:

- Review the whole change process using the Ottoway (1976) and Turrill (1985) models. Was a factor not identified in the planning stage? Are the reviews not frequent enough? Is there greater pressure than anticipated from resisters?
- Adjust the change process and replan in the light of new difficulties.
- Examine the roles that the staff occupy as these can be a source of stress (Hardy and Conway, 1978). Are they experiencing role overload (through having too much to do) or role conflict (different role expectations between the person on a job and those they work with, families, friends and so on)? The end result of either difficulty is role strain, when the stress manifests itself in the kind of physiological and psychological symptoms mentioned by Cooper *et al.* (1988).
- Identify weaknesses in the knowledge or skill of the staff which are producing role fulfilment difficulties. Provide education to fill the gap.
- Provide counselling, assertiveness training, stress awareness training or relaxation techniques for staff who are experiencing difficulties as appropriate. Within the health services, these facilities are not always available, but there has been a growing trend in recent years to develop counselling skills for key staff and to provide a counselling service in many settings. Many colleges, schools of nursing and other educational institutions provide courses in self-awareness and assertiveness and relaxation techniques. Other staff organisations, such as the Royal College of Nursing, also provide these, along with an independent counselling service.
- Ensure that steps are taken to take care of the self in the process of change, such as paying attention to eating a healthy diet, ensuring sufficient exercise and sleep is taken, finding individuals and groups

with whom problems can be shared (partners or close friends, work colleagues, supportive managers), taking time out from work and having time for yourself to pursue interests not connected with work, giving yourself breaks and treats when you need them and so on. Caring for yourself in the change process is as important if not more so than paying attention to the change strategy.

- Use team building workshops, 'away days', team meetings and social events not only to reduce stress, review progress and celebrate successes but also to build trusting and supportive relationships among the team. One group, using Manthey's (1982) (cited in Wright, 1993) 'commitment to each other' charter set about discussing how they should work together, agreed a code of good and bad behaviour and set limits and boundaries for each other in the team. It has to be noted that while writing such statements is a useful outcome, the process that people go through to achieve them, i.e. engage in honest, open dialogue with one another under the guidance of an expert facilitator, may be more important than the outcome of any written statement.

- Make use of 'networking' techniques (NHS Women's Unit, 1994) which are a useful means of sharing knowledge and experience and gaining peer support for changes at work. This might include participating in or setting up a network of people with similar interests – as occurs with the King's Fund Nursing Developments Network, The Foundation for Nursing Studies' Practice Development Nurses Forum and the great many professional groupings within the Royal College of Nursing for example. Many local initiatives occur as well as the well known groups (see addresses at the end of this chapter).

- Set up methods of staff support such as clinical supervision or mentorship schemes that encourage relationships among staff which offer mutual help and continued learning through guided reflection. A full discussion of clinical supervision is beyond the scope of this text, but a few points can be summarised as follows:

Clinical supervision – the essential principles

The profile of clinical supervision received a considerable boost with the publication of the *Vision for the future* document in 1993 (DoH, 1993). Essentially, it called upon all nurses, midwives and health visitors to explore and develop clinical supervision.

A number of authors and organisations have sought to explain the concept in more detail (Hawkins and Shohet, 1989; Butterworth and Faugier, 1992; Bishop, 1994; Butterworth and Faugier, 1994; King's Fund, 1994; Kline, 1994; UKCC, 1995).

Clinical supervision already takes place in many informal ways – for example, in the way colleagues work with each other, reflect upon and discuss their practice, and seek guidance and support from each other. In this way, nurses commonly and continuously improve expertise and the quality of patient care, and help to prevent errors and bad practice. Some professions (such as psychotherapy and midwifery) have a long history of formal methods of supervision.

Clinical supervision does not require nurses to dismiss the values of informal methods, rather to build on them and enhance them into formal approaches.

Clinical supervision – the common models

The purpose of clinical supervision is to support continuous learning by the nurse, to improve the quality of patient care, reduce the risk of errors and bad practice and provide support to reduce stress upon the nurse. So, it requires each nurse to accept their own initiatives, and the need for the support of others. Every nurse should have his or her own (at least one) clinical supervisor, a professional colleague able to support the development of his or her clinical practice. 'Support' is a key concept in clinical supervision, specifically in the development of practice, it is not concerned or to be confused with managerial supervision, counselling, disciplinary action, performance review, pay grading and other methods of staff management which already take place in various arenas. When these ideas are confused it can lead many nurses to be wary of clinical supervision, which can be viewed simply as identifying a professional coach to give guidance on our practice, not as a mechanism for managerial control or discipline.

Clinical supervision can be carried out in a variety of ways, and it is up to each nurse to choose the best model suited to his or her needs and practice context. Common models include:

1 *One-to-one supervision*
Most often this will take place between two nurses who work regularly together on the same site, perhaps meeting formally and additionally at regular intervals to discuss issues of practice development. This may be supported by the use of 'reflective diaries' – the supervisee keeping a regular account of incidents in practice which he/she wishes to discuss (Palmer *et al.*, 1994) with the supervisor. (NB – such diaries, when used, should be regarded as confidential, with the supervisee retaining control over what is or is not revealed.) It is most likely that the supervisor would be a more experienced and knowledgeable clinical nurse. For example, a primary nurse on a ward may seek 'supervision' from a colleague on the same ward who has more experience in the speciality, or perhaps from the ward manager or sister/charge nurse. Sometimes a nurse may seek supervision from his/her immediate

manager. While this can work successfully, it is important to ensure that a distinction is drawn between management and supervision. There are risks of the manager's role (which includes aspects of discipline and control) being compromised in supervision (which is concerned with guiding and coaching).

Less commonly, the nurse may seek supervision from a colleague who works in another area – although there will then be practical issues to consider such as the time and opportunity to meet in private. For most nurses, on a day-to-day (or night-by-night) basis, clinical supervision is probably best developed by being in a relationship with colleagues in the immediate setting. There will be occasions where 'time out' and private discussion time is necessary, but this will be only part of the working pattern for most nurses. Clinical supervision needs to be seen as a lived experience: an everyday part of nurses' working lives and not as a separate activity that takes place 'elsewhere' or fitted in when there is a little spare time.

2 *Group supervision*
Teams of colleagues can collectively offer supervision to each other; often meeting as a group to offer neutral support and advice. There are advantages here, in that a broader perspective can be offered, but there may be difficulties in bringing groups together. There is a need to ensure the group's work is well facilitated so that its work is constructive and objective.

3 *Networking supervision*
Sometimes it may be preferable to have a supervisor who is not an immediate working colleague, and perhaps not even in the same profession. For example, a nurse pursuing an advanced course in counselling may seek supervision from a counsellor or psychotherapist who may not be a nurse. A ward or team manager may seek support and guidance from others who may not work in the same Trust. When help external to the organisation is sought, there may be questions about who pays for the supervision, although more enlightened settings should be able to offer imaginative approaches, perhaps on a 'quid pro quo' basis. It may also be that the supervision is not to be interpreted as strictly 'clinical'. In other words, the guidance may be more concerned with the general development of a nurse's role, rather than practice expertise, e.g. a consultant nurse in one unit helps a nurse create and develop a similar role in another unit.

Each model may be used on its own, or a combination of them may be used simultaneously by any one nurse depending on his/her needs.

In developing clinical supervision at the practice level, it could be argued that as a general rule, each nurse has the right to choose his or her supervisor. However a number of factors need to be taken into consideration:

(a) The right of the supervisor to refuse to supervise. For example, if they are already fully committed to other work/supervision of others.

(b) The potential additional costs involved, for example, with the expenses and fees involved in networking supervision. The supervisor, supervisee and managers need to have clear agreements on costs and how these are to be set against specific outcomes.

(c) The supervisor and supervisee must set out the general rules and objectives of their work together and agree these in advance, e.g. frequency and provision of privacy for meetings, access to reflective diaries, options for withdrawal and agreement on confidentiality, appropriate targets to be met and so on. While the working relationship needs to be open and flexible to respond to the needs of the supervisee, it is sometimes necessary to provide evidence of practical, measurable outcomes. This may especially be so when additional costs for clinical supervision (e.g. the payment of fees to the supervisor) may have to be justified.

(d) The focus of supervision is very much on the development of the individual nurse's clinical knowledge and skills. Supervisor and supervisee need to agree on where to 'draw the line', e.g. when professional advice may extend into personal counselling, private matters and so on.

(e) The supervisor has a responsibility to ensure he/she has the skills and knowledge to supervise, to know and act upon limitations, and to take appropriate action when situations arise in the supervisor/supervisee relationships which are beyond his/her remit and the agreed ground rules.

(f) Both parties need to be committed to keeping their practice up to date and based on sound knowledge, and both need to have effective interpersonal skills to be able to work together, e.g. abiding by agreed rules, ensuring comment on practice is fair and objective, giving and receiving praise when it is due, and so on.

It is also worth noting that the supervisor needs supervision too, setting up a chain of supervision/supervisee relationships in nursing. Training for those giving and receiving supervision is necessary, so that both can give of their best and receive maximum benefit from it. The organisation has a part to play in providing this support and ongoing programmes of training are needed.

Clinical supervision aims to promote continuous learning to improve practice. It needs to be an activity present throughout our nursing lifetimes. Professional standards concerned with maintaining learning and quality of care means that it must ultimately become not an option but a lifelong requirement for all nurses.

Stress and support

Under the circumstances, it might be seen that the change process might also be a personal growth experience for those who are going through it. It must also be remembered that stressful situations at work can be exacerbated if the person is also experiencing stress in their non-working lives.

Cooper *et al.'s* (1988) stress inventory gives an indication of the extent of the issue (Table 7.2). You might wish to work with this yourself to get an idea of what your own stress levels may be like at the moment. Remember that this is only a general guide, and does not take account of stresses you may be experiencing at work because of the practice changes that are under way. If you are under stress at the moment, it might be a good idea to look at some of the ways mentioned above to reduce it. Alternatively it might be appropriate to seek the help of an expert doctor, nurse or counsellor.

If the staff and the change agents are experiencing stress, there is also a moral obligation on those who support them to examine their role. Is the education and management support that is needed being offered? Are the resources being provided? Are sufficient staff available? It is important to look at the individual's coping abilities and find ways to enhance them if stress occurs. It is also important to ensure that the situation in which the change agent and his/her colleagues must work is examined for flaws. Individuals may have weaknesses, but so do the circumstances in which they are required to work.

An area where interpersonal conflict is occasionally encountered is between the health care workers and the patient/client. The public today are becoming much better informed, through education and the media, the advent of Patient's Charters, the legal right of access to medical records and so on. In addition, many nurses and other health care workers have developed models of practice which espouse patient involvement, empowerment and advocacy. Patients and their carers are increasingly demanding that they be involved in the discussions and decisions made about themselves and their families. As professionals, health care workers are taught to assume they have more knowledge and power than their patient/client. Many nurses feel unable to cope with the stress of the new kind of relationship which emerges with the patient. Task allocation, Menzies (1960) has argued, allowed nurses to hide from the stress of a closer relationship with the patient and his or her problems. If the tasks, for example, which nurses have used as a coping strategy are removed, what are they replaced with? It is necessary to return to the points made earlier:

Table 7.2 The life stress inventory (after Cooper et al., 1988)

Place a cross (x) in the 'Yes' column for each event which has taken place in the last two years. Circle a number on the scale which best describes how upsetting the event was to you, e.g. 10 for death of spouse.

Event	Yes	Scale
Bought house		1 2 3 4 5 6 7 8 9 10
Sold house		1 2 3 4 5 6 7 8 9 10
Moved house		1 2 3 4 5 6 7 8 9 10
Major house renovation		1 2 3 4 5 6 7 8 9 10
Increased or new bank loan/mortgage		1 2 3 4 5 6 7 8 9 10
Separation from loved one		1 2 3 4 5 6 7 8 9 10
End of relationship		1 2 3 4 5 6 7 8 9 10
Got engaged		1 2 3 4 5 6 7 8 9 10
Got married		1 2 3 4 5 6 7 8 9 10
Marital problem		1 2 3 4 5 6 7 8 9 10
Awaiting divorce		1 2 3 4 5 6 7 8 9 10
Divorce		1 2 3 4 5 6 7 8 9 10
Child started school/nursery		1 2 3 4 5 6 7 8 9 10
Increased nursing responsibilities for elderly or sick person		1 2 3 4 5 6 7 8 9 10
Problems with relatives		1 2 3 4 5 6 7 8 9 10
Problems with friends/neighbours		1 2 3 4 5 6 7 8 9 10
Pet-related problems		1 2 3 4 5 6 7 8 9 10
Work-related problems		1 2 3 4 5 6 7 8 9 10
Change in nature of work		1 2 3 4 5 6 7 8 9 10
Threat of redundancy		1 2 3 4 5 6 7 8 9 10
Changed job		1 2 3 4 5 6 7 8 9 10
Made redundant		1 2 3 4 5 6 7 8 9 10
Unemployed		1 2 3 4 5 6 7 8 9 10
Retired		1 2 3 4 5 6 7 8 9 10
Financial difficulty		1 2 3 4 5 6 7 8 9 10
Insurance problem		1 2 3 4 5 6 7 8 9 10
Legal problem		1 2 3 4 5 6 7 8 9 10
Emotional or physical illness of close family or relative		1 2 3 4 5 6 7 8 9 10
Serious illness of close family or relative requiring hospitalisation		1 2 3 4 5 6 7 8 9 10
Surgical operation experienced by family member or relative		1 2 3 4 5 6 7 8 9 10
Death of spouse		1 2 3 4 5 6 7 8 9 10
Death of family member or relative		1 2 3 4 5 6 7 8 9 10
Death of close friend		1 2 3 4 5 6 7 8 9 10
Emotional or physical illness of yourself		1 2 3 4 5 6 7 8 9 10
Serious illness requiring your own hospitalisation		1 2 3 4 5 6 7 8 9 10
Surgical operation on yourself		1 2 3 4 5 6 7 8 9 10
Pregnancy		1 2 3 4 5 6 7 8 9 10
Birth of baby		1 2 3 4 5 6 7 8 9 10
Birth of grandchild		1 2 3 4 5 6 7 8 9 10
Family member left home		1 2 3 4 5 6 7 8 9 10
Difficult relationship with children		1 2 3 4 5 6 7 8 9 10
Difficult relationship with parents		1 2 3 4 5 6 7 8 9 10

Plot total score below

Low stress		High stress
1	50	100

- *Education* so that staff feel equipped to cope with a new way of doing things.
- *Support* from colleagues, and an atmosphere where both praise and sympathy are given freely, where feelings can be easily talked about, exchanged and understood.

When confronted with change at clinical level, Salvage (1988) suggests that nurses go through changes not unlike the grieving process:

- *Shock* is the first likely response; people facing change feel threatened, overwhelmed, anxious and panicky. As we know from research on patients, fear tends to close down your communication channels and limits your rational faculties.
- *Defensive retreat* can follow from an inability to cope with this shock; it is a kind of denial of it. People become negative and withdrawn, or occasionally falsely optimistic and euphoric.
- *Acknowledgement,* as in bereavement, is an important step towards acceptance, but it can involve apathy and a nostalgia for the good old days and ways just as we tend to remember the dead person in a favourable light.
- *Adaptation.* occurs if these preceding stages are worked through. When the nurse begins to mobilise her resources and abilities to meet the new situation, she begins to learn: now comes a time of challenge and growth.

With the support of the kind discussed so far in this chapter, the conflicts for staff in the change process can be minimised. The change agents and their colleagues can experience the process as a benefit not only to their client, but as a time of challenge and growth for themselves as well.

Staff changes

The implications for changing the norms and style of the workplace cannot be overestimated. Where change is minor, the effects can be minimal, but change on a grander scale such as the wholesale shifting of a group's philosophy and approach to work (for example, in shifting from an institutionalised to a personalised model of care) can produce quite dramatic effects. Ultimately, some staff will not feel able to work with the new style and, as Ottoway (1976), Martin (1984) and Wright (1985) have suggested, they may leave. While the departure of some staff may be a cause for concern (it may cost more to recruit new staff), there are several aspects to this problem. Firstly, it must be questioned whether or not it is desirable that they have left. To be blunt, is the organisation better off without them? Were they so resistant to change that it would simply not have been cost-effective to pour resources and energy into persuading them to participate? Secondly, did they leave because the change strategy was wrong and, if so, is it that which needs to be examined? Thirdly, is their leaving a cause for concern because they were considered to be among the 'better' staff? If this is the case, it may be that their qualities were overestimated, or it may be that the change has taken a new path and is not perhaps producing a change for the better.

There is a value judgement being made here, for it is assumed that change which produces a more personalised climate for both staff and patients is 'better'. There is, of course, an opposing perspective to this. The staff who have got used to the more institutionalised approach (as depicted so succinctly in Martin (1984)) may not see the new approach as 'better' but 'worse' because of the loss of the *status quo*, the old power structures, and their privileges.

We all have to make our own value judgements on these issues. However, in the final analysis, it could be argued that what nurses want is of secondary importance to what patients or clients want. If nurses believe that they know so much better than the patient or client, then the obligation is upon nursing to explain its case to them so that they can make informed choices. Certainly, if the mass of evidence that has accumulated over the years is anything to go by, patients are fairly clear about what they want from nurses – a service that is humane, friendly, informative and personal, and takes full account of their needs, and does not seek to fit them into someone else's roles. At the last, it is the patient who judges.

The client's perceptions

Almost all changes at clinical level will affect the recipient of care. In this respect, he or she provides the ultimate test of the change. The change process has to be 'sold' to the client as well as the staff. It seems that many complaints in care (DoH, 1990–96) can be attributed to the failure of the professionals to communicate adequately about why they do what they do with patients.

CASE STUDY

A family complain to the community nurse who has been helping their relative, a young woman, at home. She is disabled after a road accident, but the nurse is trying to encourage her independence by allowing her to feed herself and teaching her to do things for herself. The relatives see this as 'uncaring' as they think everything should be 'done for' their loved one. The nurse has not adequately explained her style of care to the relatives so that they will understand and share her goals.

Where nurses implement change which affects their patients or clients and those who are involved with them, then they too must be part of the change process.

Change is a personal journey

Techniques for change are relatively easy to define, but it is necessary to pause for a moment. The tendency to think of change as a linear process – a movement from A to B (such as indicated in Lewin's (1958) model of 'unfreezing', 'moving' and 'refreezing' in Chapter 3) is very strong. The success of change tends to be evaluated in terms of observable results. However, what about changes which fail? What about the reality of change for most people – that it is not so much a linear process but a complex psychological and social 'dance', constantly moving and shifting towards, around and beyond original goals? How is change perceived by the living, breathing individuals who experience it? If some changes are seen as self-evidently 'good' (e.g. the implementation of methods of patient-centred care) why is it that it seems to be so difficult to engender an uptake among the great mass of nurses?

Perhaps something remains deeply wrong in nursing and our health care systems. When something is wrong, there is a tendency to focus on systems or structures which deliver a service and this has indeed been the focus of much of change in nursing in recent years. In response to a perceived need to improve the quality of care, in the UK for example, there has been massive organisation shift in the health service, while nursing has invested huge amounts of energy in all manner of techniques ostensibly aimed at the same goal (nursing models, primary nursing, care planning, self-medication and so on). These and many other actions seem fine as far as they go, but there is more. People cry out to be treated as a whole, yet the services seem to be failing them – evidenced by the fact that over 13 million people in the UK last year, for example, opted out of the orthodox system and went to a complementary therapist. Indeed, many nurses themselves have either moved into being practitioners in these fields, or have sought to bring them into their practice. The real changes that people are seeking may be both broader and deeper than tinkering with organisations and system can meet.

The objectification of health has led us to a point of great danger for nursing. The Cartesian rational, scientific, masculine world view has struck health care worldwide this past decade as never before. As health care systems struggle to contain costs, and sometimes fall apart, there is an ever greater struggle to identify certainty amidst a sense of threat, challenge and insecurity. Worshipping at the altar of cost-effectiveness, those who control the system are increasingly sidelining nursing and many others. The knock-on effect is serious, for example:

- The tendency to justify 'rationing' of health care (under the guise of prioritising) and to apportion it accordingly to the deserving and the undeserving (the latter group usually consisting of elderly people, the chronically ill, the disabled and so on).
- The use of language as euphemism to justify these decisions, e.g. 'prioritising', 'downsizing', 're-engineering'.
- The focus on actions which are observable and measurable (the instrumental (Benner, 1984) skills). Yet so much of nursing is 'invisible' (Lawler, 1991). However, if it cannot be measured, the risk is that it will not be paid for in a system which recognises only tasks, measurable actions and outcomes.
- Within nursing itself the objectification seems to be producing a class of people who subscribe to the view that the rationalist–scientific model is all that matters. In some realms of nursing academia for example, in order to appear rational and scientific, to gain social acceptance within this world view, the elite have so distanced themselves not only from the reality of nursing practice, but indeed its very heart, that they damage nursing rather than encourage it. Sogyal Rinpoche (1992) summarises this view:

Our contemporary education indoctrinates us in the glorification of doubt, has created in fact what could almost be called a religion or theology of doubt, in which to be seen to be intelligent we have to be seen to doubt everything, to always point to what's wrong and rarely to ask what's right or good, cynically to denigrate all inherited ideals and philosophies, or any theory that is done in simple goodwill or an innocent heart.

This unfolding process (and it is still unfolding) is deeply rooted in the professional nursing psyche, and is the end product of our own lack of confidence and certainty in our own centre, our own values. 'Things fall apart; the centre cannot hold' writes the poet W.B. Yeats. When things fall apart, unsure of our own centre, we look to the narcissistic mirror offered by others to bring certainty into an uncertain world. Science, technology, reason appear to offer these certainties, a centre which holds. However, this model is only half adequate for nursing, so much else in nursing relies upon meaning, intuition, feelings, not so much upon what nurses 'do' with patients, but how we 'are' with them – our true being.

But what is this 'true' being that is the nurse? What is this centre which needs to hold? To consider these questions it means that we as nurses have to look internally, rather than externally. Perhaps our focus on external change (form), giving the impression that we are improving things, is a sign not so much of our success but of our insecurity, our inability to face what is really going on inside and what we really need to deal with. The external activities may be not so much evidence of our success in improving care, but of denial. We look to the outer because the inner is too difficult and painful to bear. However, without a sound basis of inner centredness and certainty the outer lacks substance, feels un-centred and is dehumanised. It contains the head but not the heart of nursing and fails as a result. The outer manifestations of nursing may be taking place, but several things are missing. People can feel cared for, but not cared about, and enough of them sense this to turn away from us (and enough nurses sense this to move into other ways of being, e.g. becoming a complementary therapist), in order to be in a situation where they can express themselves.

Studies have found high levels of 'co-dependence' among nurses (Snow and Willard, 1989) and exposed the myths and truths about nursing; for example:

Table 7.3 Myths and truths of nursing

Myths	Truths
Nurses know how to look after themselves and should be healthy.	The truth is, nurses suffer from low back pain, chronic colitis and other gastric disturbances, chronic urinary tract infections, migraine headaches, high blood pressure, hypo and hyperglycemia, skin disease, depression and other stress-related disorders.
Nurses know about, understand and treat the diseases of addiction and, therefore, should not have them.	80+ per cent of nurses may be co-dependent and often mediate the pain of their disease with alcohol, drugs, food, sex, spending, gambling, serial unhappy relationships and more. Nurses are just as addicted, if not more so, than the general population.
Nurses live to care for others and should love the rewards they get from their work.	A nurse's work is often demeaning, depressing, gruelling, discounting and demanding – and nurses do burn out.
Nurses are natural caregivers, trained to work with others, therefore, should have excellent parenting skills.	Nurses often bring fatigue, anger, shame, fear, pain, and job and financial worries into their home environments and have little energy for effective parenting.
Nurses should be spiritually inspired healers.	Nurses are required to accept physicians, other nurse colleagues and institutions as gods, and they come to believe that they, too, can be in control. Spiritual practices and the art of healing are effectively shut down from this perspective.

Supporting this view have been the recent alarms raised in the UK about the high stress levels, sickness and suicide rates among nurses. There are many factors which can be attributed to these phenomena, and there can be little doubt that inhospitable managerial cultures, heavy workloads and so on play a major part. Meanwhile, the trend towards more patient-centred care and the decline of task allocation are leading nurses on to ever more intimate (stressful?) relationships with patients. However, the malaise may run deeper than this. Perhaps the greatest change we need to embark upon in nursing is not so much the 'external', but the internal, to heal the 'wounded healers' (Moyers, 1993). Dossey (1995), for example, argues that:

At the root of the problem lies the fact that we, as a culture, have turned our collective back on healing ... ignoring the role of consciousness, soul, spirit, and meaning – stock items in the arsenal of authentic healers – we have birthed a malaise that permeates not just the healing profession, but our entire society.

Thomas' studies (1976) of medical students indicated that:

Students whose psychological tests showed that they could not externalise their feelings – those who kept things bottled up inside – developed fatal cancers in later life at an increased incidence.

Dossey (1991) response that:

The implications are chilling. Medical schools in general foster the internalisation of feelings – the 'I can take it' attitude in which one never complains, no matter how difficult the situation.

Salvage (1985) and many others have argued that exactly the same phenomenon occurs in nursing schools – in relation both to the experiences of practice and theory work in the college of nursing.

Of course, this is a contentious territory. It is not politically correct, in the UK for example, to suggest that nurses are not coping, rather that we are at the leading edge of change and forging ahead with the agenda. Furthermore, the 'internal' is seen as too private – leave well alone, don't disturb the defence mechanisms. This ostrich-like syndrome (itself a form of denial) assumes that there is no problem and that nurses can cope.

While not denying the need for continued external change, it may be that an area of change we must now also face in nursing is internal. Some of the strategies are relatively straightforward, for example, in terms of providing support for nurses at a wider organisational level (Snow and Willard, 1989; NASS, 1992), amongst the team at local/unit level and through personal strategies such as meditation, exercise, counselling, time out and so on. More enlightened organisations are moving in this direction. Not least because investing in staff in this way is seen as cost-effective.

A second area of attention is to change the current focus in the rational–scientific and to bring these into balance with the intuitive. This is not either/or but both: 'Our second perspective is that when nurses rely *solely* on factual, linear, research-guided models of care, they fail to integrate intuitive principles that have been known for centuries and that complete the healing process. These intuitive principles are feelings, ways of knowing answers to problems that either are not provable or defy scientific law. When applied to Western healing practices, alternative healing methods – certain forms of touch, energy balancing, psychic skills – often make no sense. Yet they work' (Snow and Willard, 1989). Thus a rebalancing of healing skills, of masculine and feminine perspectives, is seen as essential to the restoration of healing in health care generally, and nursing specifically.

A third element may be much more problematic for many. An adherence to objective, rationalist values has another knock-on effect – a denial of the spiritual basis of our practice. This is best characterised in the nursing process, where we ask the patient 'what religion are you?' – then hand the matter over to the minister. Spiritual needs are thereby glossed over, and yet: 'Without faith in a power greater than ourselves – greater than our parents – we have difficulty with relationships that operate on other than surface levels. We often are afraid to be honest with ourselves or to believe in the honesty of another's love. Further, without spirituality, we find it impossible to believe in something better for ourselves. The cynical messages – from society, our families, our colleagues, our friends – that tell us to settle for less than trust, honesty, and intimacy in relationships nourish the delusion that we *can't* have a relationship on a deep level ... A relationship without spirituality is a frightening place to be. Spirituality assures us we are not alone. Spirituality assures us we do not have to be in control of others – what they do, what they feel, what they think. Spirituality gives us the courage to trust, to be honest and, therefore, vulnerable, and to live in acceptance of ourselves and others' (Snow and Willard, 1989). Thus, nursing values and actions based entirely upon humanistic, atheistic, rationalistic thinking may be an inadequate base to create that certain centre for each nurse. In the process of managing change and dealing with the stress and strain of it, many nurses find themselves searching for deeper meaning, connection and understanding in what we do.

The case studies discussed in the previous chapter illustrate how the change process was as much an inner personal journey as well as an outer one of changing the system.

Unfortunately, there is a tendency to look for old certainties when fear stalks us. Fears about the future of nursing and the loss of its values base, have led some (Bradshaw, 1994) to call for a return to orthodox, Christian, almost fundamentalist beliefs. This, however, denies the pluralistic nature of the modern world, and how a new paradigm, which embraces the spiritual, is emerging as the millennium draws to a close. Carey (1991), for example, argues: 'To choose religious or ideological dogmatism in the name of freedom is as foolish as for a jailed man to exercise his right to remain in prison'. The answer may therefore lie not in a religious or dogmatic revival in nursing (even Florence Nightingale said 'The law of God, it seems, is against repetition' (Poovey, 1991)), but in a spiritual one – but the journey starts 'here', 'in the heart'.

Enormous amounts of attention are paid to changing systems, structures, organisations. It needs to be remembered that this may be only half the story. There is a need to ensure that relationships are right as well – with ourselves, with our colleagues, with our organisations. We need to be, however, not just in right relationships with each other, but also with ourselves, and that means reviewing, re-energising and revitalising who we are and what we do, how we exist in the world, what meaning and value we bring to our work. Thomas (1983), for example, believed that: 'We do not know enough about ourselves. We are ignorant about how we work, about where we fit in and most of all about the enormous, imponderable system of life in which we are embedded as working parts'.

In order to enter into right relationships with others, we may first have to enter into a right relationship with ourselves and that may transcend the very limited scientific view of what we are as human beings, and re-examine and incorporate spiritual values. Everyone who has contributed to this book has found that participation and change has meant a personal transformation as well as an organisational one. In fact, it could be argued that as we mature and grow as individuals into 'right relationships' with ourselves, then the things we seek to achieve externally are more likely to be successful. The outer falls into place when the inner is in harmony.

Change agents may become laggards too!

CASE STUDY

A group of student nurses is discussing their experiences in a unit with the clinical nurse specialist. They have a number of complaints and weaknesses to bring out. The response of the senior nurse is to become defensive. 'You've no idea what it was like here years ago. I was brought in to make things better and we've made immense changes at great personal cost I can tell you! Of course, I don't expect you to appreciate all that, you don't remember how difficult it was in those days.'

The above example is the classic trap for the change agents. Resentment may occur when people still seem to want to change things. But, as was noted earlier, permanence is dead! The desire to change things will emerge continually, but at a cost to the change agent who may have accumulated so much power so as to become the conservative in the organisation.

There is a scene from a famous TV series of the 1960s and 70s, *Monty Python's Flying Circus* (1974), which mirrors this perfectly. Four 'old codgers' discuss their past, each trying to outdo the other in portraying how much hardship they endured, and how much easier the youngsters of today have it!

Without continuous education, moving on, opportunities for reflection, the guidance of trusted colleagues, new challenges, exposure to performance review, appraisal and evaluation then those who have changed things may become complacent. The 'wallpaper effect' occurs; having visited a place so often, the blemishes and faults ceased to be noticed. Sometimes it takes a visitor to point them out. The trajectory of change has no terminus, only regular stops along the way to an infinite destination. Keeping the system and ourselves open to constant challenge and change helps to prevent complacency and resistance to change setting in.

'Tall poppy' syndrome

Faugier (1993) has described the 'tall poppy' syndrome; that is the tendency in nursing for individuals who challenge and change things and stand out from the crowd to be greeted with fear, hostility and envy rather than praise and encouragement. Using an Australian analogy of fields of corn where the poppies are cut down because they grow taller and are bright and stand out. Likewise, she argued, this is what happens in nursing which tends to have disdain for bright, articulate personalities who dare to be different. Sheehan and Wright (1995) have identified a similar process affecting groups associated with change such as NDUs. It is characterised by criticism, undermining of credibility and authority, blaming and 'backstabbing'. It might be expected that those who change nursing for the better would be celebrated, and while this happens, the negative tall poppy syndrome is at work too. It is closely associated with fears of change and a sign of professional and personal immaturity that seeks to denigrate the work of others rather than celebrate it, but that is not to underestimate its impact upon those at the receiving end who can feel hurt and threatened. Often they can be the subject of all kinds of rumour and innuendo (you've only succeeded because you've got more money/time/staff/ support from the manager etc!). For every person who acclaims their successes, there seems to be another who seeks to bring them down. Those involved in change can help reduce some of the worst effects by:

- making sure that all the staff are aware of this phenomenon so that they are prepared for it when it happens;
- keeping the place where change is happening open and receptive to others, through visitors' programmes, open days, study sessions, briefing meetings and so on;
- making a point of approaching and visiting other individuals and sites to explain about the changes;
- making information available through publications, newsletters, information sheets and so on;
- offering help and guidance to others, sharing expertise and information;
- discussing the changes at various meetings and policy making groups to ensure it is on the agenda and maintaining awareness of the reality of what is going on;
- ensuring that rumour and misinformation is countered either directly or through the media, supportive managers and so on;
- using a change strategy that involves as many people as possible, and prevents any team members from feeling excluded.

Thus a number of steps can be taken to alleviate the worst effects of the 'tall poppy' syndrome, although it has to be remembered that this phenomenon is deeply rooted in nursing and until nursing changes its culture completely, will continue to be present and an issue to deal with.

Financial implications

The process of change may exert financial pressures on the organisation, at the same time it may also save money. In times of economic stringency in health care, nurses are required more and more to put a good case forward if we wish to change things. If it is likely to save money, all well and good. The idea may be less well received if there is a higher cost implication. Sometimes changes which may make a demand for more money can be suppressed, and this is perhaps an understandable response by those who bear the responsibility of controlling the purse strings. However, the quality of life of staff and patients cannot be measured in terms of cost alone.

Sometimes costs can be met within existing resources, for example, by converting posts within a given staffing budget. One group of nurses in an intensive care unit carried out a work study to evaluate how much time was spent on secretarial and other non-nursing duties, and were able to use the results to make a case for secretarial help. The money was found within the existing budget by reallocating the nursing budget accordingly. In addition, once the unit secretary was in post, more support was then available to nursing staff with the preparation and writing up of other studies and projects in which they were involved. In other settings, funds might be sought from external sources, such as charitable trusts, making approaches to a health authority or seeking research and development monies from various national and regional organisations. Even so, with any development there is often a heavy reliance upon the support of the staff in the organisation both to direct resources appropriately and to give the commitment. While Purdy and Wright (1988) have identified ways in which small units can set up nursing bursaries to identify external sources of money, to generate income so that the limited resources of the organisation can be applied to the full, often, it is not the grand schemes which cause the biggest difficulties, but the day-to-day concern over payments to sustain the change process, for example:

- supporting staff development, attendance at courses, conferences, etc;
- providing equipment involved in the change, e.g. stationery, computers;
- buying in teaching, consultancy and research expertise from other agencies;
- use of staff time, either for teaching or development purposes: both teacher and taught will not be making their full contribution to the immediate service needs of the organisation;
- paying for resources to assist the learning/development process, e.g. providing books, journals, teaching equipment, as well as accommodation, furnishings, secretarial support and so on.

The list of potential costs can be enormous. Sometimes it can be costed out fairly precisely as in applications for research grants or development monies while at other times the true cost can remain hidden or difficult to calculate.

However, where 'money' is a crucial factor, it seems that the following choices might need to be considered:

1 Can the change be managed within the existing resources?

2 Even if there is an initial cost, might the change eventually produce changes which may save money in the long term? (If so, how can this be demonstrated? Does the manager need a balance sheet of hard facts?)

3 What external sources of finance and support are available such as trust funds, research grants, bursaries? There are possibilities here worth exploring:

- Check if the organisation itself has trust funds/bursaries available for assistance.
- Contact the library or local authority for information on organisations willing to support innovations (e.g. the Guide to Company Giving (Directory of Social Change, 1986)).There are several directories available listing charities and other bodies and stipulating what kind of work they will support.
- Check local/national/nursing press for organisations offering assistance (e.g. the Nightingale Fund, the Smith and Nephew Foundation, and so on).
- Investigate educational establishments for guidelines sources/for application for grants.
- Contact appropriate professional bodies, institutes, health service organisations, etc. for avenues of funding.
- Consider ways of raising funding locally, e.g. sponsorship schemes, conferences, consultancy fees, local support groups (e.g. League of Friends), fundraising activities, getting support through the local press. Using networks of friends/local contacts who may be able to identify a possible sponsor.

These and more possibilities can be explored to support the costs of the change. Much depends on the size of the scheme to be pursued, the length of time it will need, and the abilities of many individuals concerned with it to draw upon their entrepreneurial skills to raise money.

Everything has its price, and changing nursing practice is no exception. Perhaps the most important aspect in this respect is the acceptance by the organisation as a whole, and those persons within it, that change is a continuous and acceptable normal part of its legitimate activities. When the culture of the organisation accepts change at this level, then the opportunity is so much greater for other parts of the change process to flow from it and through it.

When faced with the comment, 'We cannot afford to change', the riposte might well be, 'Can we afford not to?'.

References

Bailey, R.D. 1985 *Coping with stress in caring.* Blackwell Scientific Publications, Oxford.

Benner, P. 1984 *From novice to expert.* Addison Wesley, New York.

Bishop, V. 1994 Clinical supervision for an accountable profession. *Nursing Times* **90** (39), 35–37.

Bradshaw, A. 1994 *Lighting the lamp.* Scutari, London.

Butterworth, T. and Faugier, J. 1992 *Clinical supervision and mentorship in nursing.* Chapman & Hall, London.

Butterworth, C.A. and Faugier, J. 1994 *Clinical supervision in nursing,* *midwifery and health visiting. A briefing paper.* The School of Nursing Studies, University of Manchester.

Carey, K. 1991 *The third millennium.* Harper, San Francisco.

Cherniss, C. 1980 *Staff burnout: job stress in the human services.* Sage, London.

Cooper, C., Cooper, R. and Eaten, L. 1988 *Living with stress.* Penguin, Harmondsworth.

Department of Health 1993 *A vision for the future.* DOH, London.

Department of Health 1996 *The Health Service Ombudsman Reports.* DoH, London.

Directory of Social Change 1986 *A guide to company giving.* Bath Press, Bath.

Dossey, L. 1995 Whatever happened to healers? *Alternative Therapies* **1** (5), 6–13.

Faugier J. 1993 Tall poppies. *Nursing Times* **88** (50), 20.

Hardy, M.E. and Conway, M.E. 1978 *Role theory: perspectives for health professionals.* Appleton Century Croft, New York.

Hawkins, P. and Shohet, R. 1989 *Supervision in the helping professions.* Open University Press, Milton Keynes.

King's Fund Centre 1994 *Clinical supervision: an executive summary.* King's Fund Centre, London.

Kohner, N. 1994 *Clinical supervision in practice.* King's Fund Centre, London.

Lazarus, M. and Lannier, R. 1981 Stress related transactions between person and environment. In: Dervin, L.A. and Lewis, M. (Eds), *Perspectives in interpersonal psychology.* Plenum, New York.

Lawler, J. 1991 *Behind the screens.* Churchill Livingstone, Edinburgh.

Lewin, K. 1958 The group reaction and social change. In: Macoby, E. (Ed). *Readings in social psychology.* Holt, Rinehart and Winston, London.

Manthey, M. 1994 Commitment to each other. Cited in Wright, S.G. 1993 *My patient – my nurse.* Scutari, London.

Martin, J.P. 1984 *Hospitals in trouble.* Blackwell, Oxford.

Menzies, I. 1960 A case study on the functioning of social systems as a defence against anxiety. *Human Relations* **13**, 95–121.

Monty Python's Flying Circus 1974 *Four Yorkshiremen.* Monty Python Charisma Records, London.

Moyers, B. 1993 Wounded Healers. *Parabola* **18** (1), 21–30.

National Association of Staff Support 1992 *A Charter for staff support.* NASS, Woking.

NHS Womens Unit 1994 *Networking.* DoH, London.

Ottoway, R.N. 1976 A change strategy to complement new norms, new styles and new environment in the work organisation. *Personnel Review* **5**(1), 1318.

Palmer, A., Burns, S. and Bulman, C. 1994 *Reflective practice in nursing.* Blackwells, Oxford.

Poovey, M. (Ed.) 1991 Nightingale, F. *Cassandra! – suggestions for thought.* Pickering, London.

Purdy, E. and Wright, S.G. 1988 If I were a rich nurse. *Nursing Times* **84**(41), 368.

Salvage, J. 1985 *The politics of nursing.* Heinemann, London.

Salvage, J. 1988 *Facilitating model-based nursing.* Paper given at Gateshead Nursing Models Conference. Unpublished.

Sheehan, A. and Wright, S.G. 1995 Cut flowers. *Nursing Standard* **9**(35) 46–47.

Snow, C. and Willard, P. 1989 *I'm dying to take care of you.* Professional Counsellor Books, Redmond WA.

Sogyal, R. 1992 *The Tibetan book of living and dying.* Ryder Books, London.

Thomas, C.B. 1976 Precursors of premature disease and death: the predictive potential of habits and family attitudes. *Annals of Internal Medicine* **85**, 653–658.

Thomas, L. 1983 *The medusa and the snail.* Bantam, New York.

Thomson, R. 1977 *The psychology of thinking.* Penguin, Harmondsworth.

Turrill, T. 1985 Change and innovation. *A Challenge for the NHS.* Management Series 10. Institute of Health Service Management, London.

UKCC (1995) *Initial position statement on clinical supervision for nursing and health visiting.* UKCC, London.

Wright, S.G. 1985 Change in nursing: the application of change theory to practice. *Nursing Practice* **1** (2), 85–91.

Wright, S.G. 1989 *Changing nursing practice* (1st edn.) Arnold, London.

Useful addresses of organisations cited in this chapter

NHS Women's Unit
Department of Health
Eileen House
80–94 Newington Causeway
London SE1 6EF.

Royal College of Nursing
20 Cavendish Square
London W1M OAB.

Health Visitors' Association
50 Southwark Street
London SE1 1UN.

Royal College of Midwives
15 Mansfield Street
London W1M 0BE.

Unison
20 Grand Depot Road
London SE18 6SF.

King's Fund Nursing Developments Network
11–13 Cavendish Square
London W1M 0AN.

Foundation of Nursing Studies
130 Buckingham Palace Road
London SW1 9SA.

8 Evaluation

Dirk Keyzer with Stephen Wright

Introduction
Quantitative or qualitative methods: which do we choose?
Performance indicators
The who of evaluation
Anatomy of an innovation

We seem to exist in a hazardous time Driftin' along here through space;
Nobody knows just how we began, Or how far we've gone in the race.

Ben King, *Evolution*

Introduction

The complex nature of nursing in its social and organisational setting makes it difficult to define the human activity of evaluation in simple terms. Given that the social and organisational role of the nurse is so diverse and complex, it follows that any attempt to evaluate the service provided, or any change in any part of it, will be problematic. This may be the reason why the concept of evaluation is so difficult for many nurses to understand and why the term is used to describe a wide range of activities from assessment to the carrying out of research methodologies.

Within the context of the nursing process, assessment is defined by McFarlane and Castledine (1982) as the identification of actual and potential patient problems on which the plan of care is based. Evaluation, as defined by these writers, is the process whereby actual patient outcomes are compared with the desired outcomes stated in the care plan. Thus, evaluation may be viewed as the collection and interpretation of information, by formal or informal means, to aid defensible decision-making. It is also helpful to view evaluation as a continuum, with the making of value judgements at one end, and the rigorous methodologies of research at the other. In daily practice, we can find ourselves at any point along this continuum in the evaluation of our own performance, the quality of care received by the patient, or the service offered by the organisation.

Quantitative or qualitative methods: which do we choose?

Friend and Hayward (1986) and Lathleen *et al.* (1986) in their separate brief discussions on the evaluation of change in nursing outline two approaches. These approaches are categorised as: the quantitative or positivist model, and the qualitative or realist model. Like the change strategies discussed in Chapter 2, these approaches to evaluation are based on different and sometimes opposing assumptions.

The quantitative model is based on the assumption that scientific knowledge is obtainable only from data that can be directly experienced and verified between independent observers. Lathleen *et al.* (1986) argue that this approach is characterised by its commitment to an empirical base for scientific knowledge and to a notion of cause. The underlying assumptions of this approach are that its methods have a neutral value and that people can be studied as inert objects. The possibility that individuals and groups may initiate actions of their own accord, or in response to the complex interactions within groups, is overlooked in this model.

The purpose of the quantitative approach is to produce statements about causal relationships between discrete variables. This is achieved by isolating them from their natural surroundings and by artificially manipulating one or more of these variables. Statistical sampling is used to ensure that the cases studied reflect the population as a whole. This model has been widely used in the physical, biological and social sciences. It is the one most nurses will be familiar with through their basic and post basic education programmes and in their collaboration with medical colleagues' research programmes in clinical practice. However, like any methodologies, quantifiable approaches have their limitations, not least the current view arising from the field of quantum physics, that true objectivity is impossible. It seems that what is observed is influenced in may subtle ways by the observer (Sheldrake, 1995).

Quantitative methods are widely used in the current manpower planning programmes initiated by nurses throughout the country. Examples of these include the ratings scales developed to determine patient dependency such as the Aberdeen system, the Naylor–Horne model for calculating the demand for and supply of nurses, the competency rating scales used to evaluate the process of nursing, and a wide range of patient questionnaires and other systems distributed by the ward, unit or institution to determine patient satisfaction with the care received.

In contrast to the quantitative approach, qualitative methodologies focus on the subject's perceptions of the degree of change achieved that determines the success or failure of the innovation (Keyzer, 1985). Its methodologies tend towards internal rather than external evaluation. Parlett and Hamilton (1972) argued that to evaluate the changes brought about by innovations in complex human organisations the researcher has to leave his or her laboratory and study the group dynamics in the reality of the group's life. In this way, the qualitative approach acknowledges the emotional and social components of human behaviour ignored by the quantitative methods. By taking into account the effect individuals and organisational factors have on the behaviour of individuals and groups, the qualitative approach enables the evaluator to reinforce observation with discussion and background enquiry to promote an informed account of the innovation in action (Parlett and Hamilton, 1972). This approach has now become much more widely used in nursing research and evaluation, although it still encounters problems with the dominant quantitative methodology in use in the medical/health care field and is often accused of lacking 'rigour' and scientific credibility.

The question asked in the heading of this section was related to which of these approaches would most suit the evaluation of change. The answer to that question is both. Black's (1991) study, for example, used a rich matrix of both methods from leavers' surveys to patient death rates, from interviews with staff so that they could tell their story to rating scales in questionnaires. The result produced a detailed and insightful account of change in a nursing setting. Thus, in the reality of the work environment it is likely that both quantitative and qualitative methods will be used. There are no hard and fast rules to be applied and much will depend on what is to be evaluated and why it is being carried out. For example, if the organisation wants to know the numbers of nurses required to meet the patient's needs for care, it may use quantitative methods to calculate the demand for and supply of nurses, but semi-structured interviews that is qualitative methods, to determine the patient's needs for care and satisfaction with the care received. It must also be remembered that in discussing the efficiency of change attention should also be drawn to the quality of the desired outcomes.

Performance indicators

The term 'performance indicator' can be defined as a gauge or device for measuring an institution's and/or its component parts' level of success in achieving the objectives set for it in the organisation's strategic and operational plans. Performance indicators are tools which assist the nurse in evaluation of the service offered to the public. Such an evaluation is orientated more towards the whole system rather than individuals who work in it. Appraisal of staff and the manner in which they utilise available resources are nevertheless part of the review of the whole system. Reid (1986) suggested that performance indicators could be considered as pointers that draw attention to many functions which include the use of resources and clinical activity, and cover the dimensions of economy, efficiency, accessibility and achievement of policy. Standards of care can be set and audited to judge how a particular nursing function is performing in relation to what is deemed a desirable standard. Benchmarking, clinical audit, evidence-based practice and value-for-money exercises have all emerged as ways of making judgements about the effectiveness of services, i.e. evaluating them. Hospital 'league tables' began to emerge in the mid 1990s in response to government policy and in an attempt to make more information available to the public about the performance of a particular trust. As yet, this policy does not apply to the private sector. The tables themselves often reveal very little other than raw statistics, and there is much room for improvement. There may be information about success rates in relation to a particular surgeon, but this may say little about whether that surgeon is dealing with the more difficult cases that affect the results. Without the qualitative context, the data may be open to misinterpretation. Furthermore much of the data released tends to focus on medical interventions. Potential patients may wish to know what the death rate or re-admission rate is like in their local hospital, but the hospital's record on staff education and skills development, dealing with complaints or quality of therapeutic relationships may be of equally valid significance. Likewise, clinical audit has tended to focus very much on medical activity, and only recently is this being addressed to bring nursing and other disciplines more into the equation (Malby, 1996).

The who of evaluation

Identifying who is asking for the evaluation can help us clarify where the demand for information is coming from and the nature of the data to be gathered. For example, when a doctor asks for an evaluation of the patient's progress, the data required are most likely to be concerned with the patient's response to medical intervention. If, however, a nurse asks for an evaluation of the same patient, the data required would reflect that patient's response to nursing interventions. For the nurse manager, the same patient's needs for care may be translated into information related to the number of nursing hours needed to provide care and, hence, the number of nurses needed to staff the clinical areas. Thus different information about the same patient and his or her progress is required to meet the needs of the different groups providing input to the service offered. Identifying the source of the demand for information can determine what is to be evaluated, the method used to collect the data, and who is going to interpret the information provided.

An identification of the source of the demand for information can assist in describing the focus of the evaluation. Therefore, the 'who' of the evaluation can determine the object or subject of the process. For example, the teacher may focus attention on the student's ability to correlate theory to practice in the clinical area whereas the charge nurse may view the same student in terms of the skill mix required to meet the demands for care in the ward, and the nurse manager may look at the same student in terms of the cost of the placement in the unit. In this way, the teacher would focus on the student's problem-. solving skills, the charge nurse on his or her clinical expertise and place in the nursing team, and the manager on his or her salary in relation to the overall budget for the service. A different source can mean a different focus for the evaluation.

The source of the demand for the evaluation can also identify who will be making the judgement on the adequacy of the information gathered. This is of critical importance in that evaluation is about making value judgements on the worth of the service provided. The setting of goals for health services, the nursing service and its education programmes is a reflection of the values held by the various groups controlling and providing the service. In their everyday experience of the nursing service, patients, doctors, nurses, accountants, teachers and other groups make their subjective and objective evaluations of the service offered. Each of these groups evaluates the service from their own value systems and priorities for the service. Doctors have for a long time insisted on peer review, that is the quality of medical care evaluated from a medical perspective. That does not necessarily imply that what medicine accepts as a quality service will be accepted by the consumer of that service, or indeed by those who work with them.

Any evaluation of the nursing service and education programme based on the expectations of one group may be rejected by another. Thus an evaluation of the education programme by nurse teachers may be considered to be invalid by another organisational group whose value system differs from that of teachers. Kitson (1986) has argued that any evaluation of the quality of care provided by nurses should be viewed in the light of nursing values, that is, a nursing perspective. The same argument could also be made for an evaluation of the nursing education system. One of the problems in taking a nursing perspective is that nursing has for so long been dominated by the medical profession that little attention has been paid to nursing values by nurses. Previous reviews of the nursing service in research studies have been influenced by the nurse's need to approach the subject matter through the eyes of other disciplines, such as sociology. The current move towards the implementation of nursing models in practice and education, together with the greater access to higher education for nurses, should overcome this problem of agreement on what is and what is not a proper nursing perspective and the value placed on clinical practice and education by nurses.

It is also important to remember that values do not remain constant but change over time. What is held to be a quality service today may be rejected tomorrow. There are many examples of how nursing values have changed in recent times. Examples of the changes in nursing values are: the rejection of routinised care in favour of planned care; the demand for student status for learners; and a greater willingness to take the patients' perceptions of their needs for care into account. Whether or not the service provided by nurses meets the profession's expectations of the service depends greatly on the value it attaches to clinical practice and education. These professional values may be a reflection of the wider social values expressed by the population. In defining the source of the evaluation, the nurse takes deliberate steps to describe the value system to be used in making decisions about the outcomes of the review and the acceptability of the information gathered.

Some of the difficulties of evaluation will now be illustrated by examining another case study. The case study looks at some of the major factors in one setting where a change agent was employed to specifically alter an established care of the elderly setting.

CASE STUDY

One method to attempt to reduce the theory and practice gap in nursing, and its consequences, is to create joint appointments to produce a job which encompasses both teaching and practice. The teaching often takes place in a separate setting, such as a School of Nursing or University, and the practice (which may also involve some 'clinical' teaching in a particular ward or in the community, where the postholder takes direct responsibility for giving patient care).

In one project (Wilkinson, 1983; Wright, 1983) the joint appointment role was developed specifically as a change agent, not only to affect nurse education, but also nursing practice. The 'Learning Climate' (Orton, 1981) on the care of the elderly unit could not be refashioned until the practice setting had

CASE STUDY - Contd

been changed from an institutionalised approach to a patient-centred one. Thus it may be argued that in order to produce a learning climate (i.e. student-centred environment) then the clinical setting must first and foremost be patient-centred. This would then match the ethos of the School of Nursing which tends to teach nursing as a patient-centred activity). The job description for the joint appointments specifically incorporated these aims, and clearly designated the joint appointees as change agents, not only in producing an alternative educational model, but in changing practice as well.

The setting originally chosen was a ward of 25 patients (male) dealing with acute medical problems of the over 65s. It was part of a unit of four wards and one day hospital (50 places). Significant changes took place in nursing practice. It is upon these changes that this study concentrates and in particular the methods by which they were achieved.

Change strategies

It is one thing to create a role with a specific brief of being a change agent, quite another to see the desired changes brought about. The choice of setting was quite deliberate, being a ward in an old workhouse building with facilities and an environment somewhat unsuited to the type of care being given. There was a heavy dependence on untrained nursing auxiliaries to meet staffing levels, and great difficulty in recruiting trained staff to the ward in particular and to the unit in general. There was an emphasis on task-centred care and a 'getting through the work' approach (Clark, 1978), producing a ritualised and institutionalised style of nursing. Coser (1963), Wells (1980) and Miller and Gwynne (1972), for example, have illustrated the detrimental effect that such settings have upon patients and carers. In this instance, a specific change agent role (the joint appointment) was created to concurrently affect both care and learning.

It is possible to bring about change in people's behaviour by a direct authoritarian approach, i.e. by telling them how to do things differently. Rogers' (1969) influential philosophy, however, suggests that there are risks in this model. When the authority moves on, or becomes less effective, then there is a danger that a reversion to old norms and values takes place. Change can only become permanent if the desired values and attitudes have become a permanent part of the people in the care setting. One institutional framework can be broken down, but an alternative resilient framework must take its place if the changes are not to be swept away when the change agent departs.

For alternative goals and values to be reached for people to come to a different view of their world, the egalitarian strategy is a necessary tool. Kuhn

(1970) sees knowledge as set in paradigms of ideas about the world. When a paradigm is in conflict with new knowledge it enters a state of crisis; a new way of looking at things is set up and a new paradigm established. An example of this would be the change in our concept of caring for and preventing pressure sores once our knowledge as to the cause of them had been developed.

Lewin's (1958) classic change theory defines 'no change' as a 'quasistationary equilibrium . . . a state comparable to that of a river which flows with a given velocity in a given direction during a certain time interval'. He describes social changes as comparable to a change in the velocity and the direction of that river, and sees the change process as having three basic steps (see additional detail in Chapter 3):

- _Unfreezing_ when the motivation to create some sort of change occurs, the impetus for this comes from three possible mechanisms:
  - (a) _lack of confirmation_ or disconfirmation, i.e. the awareness of a need for change because expectations have not been met.
  - (b) _inducing of guilt or anxiety,_ i.e. uncomfortable feelings because of some action or lack of action.
  - (c) _psychological safety_ when a former obstacle to change has been removed.
- _Moving_ in which change is planned and initiated where cognitive redefinition occurs to look at the problem from a new perspective either through 'identification' or 'scanning' (the former solution provided by a knowledgeable peer; the latter solution found in a variety of sources).
- _Refreezing_ in which change is integrated into the value system and stabilised into a new equilibrium.

In order to 'unfreeze' existing norms, and 'move' the staff to 'refreeze' into new norms, a tool to do the job is required. Many alternatives are available, and producing change in nursing is often a designated role for many practitioners, managers and educators. In this instance, however, a new role was created whose prime function was to change existing patterns of care and learning. In addition, a role emerged which straddled four diverse fields of nursing (practice, management, teaching, research) and which was financed and supported by two structures in nursing that are normally quite separately organised, namely the education and service sectors. The support and commitment of the managers in these sectors was to be a crucial factor in enabling the joint appointees to fully develop their role as change agents.

Ottoway's (1976) taxonomy (described in detail in Chapter 3) identifies a number of change agent types, and perhaps the joint appointees in this particular scheme had elements of all three, being change generators, implementors and adopters. However, as Salvage (1985) has noted, the experiment took place in a very ordinary setting. The posts were created out of existing budgets and existing staffing levels, with no special facilities or added benefits provided. Wilkinson (1984), as the Director of Nurse Education involved, has pointed out that she and the Director of Nursing Services deliberately took this approach. If similar changes were to be adopted elsewhere in the division, then resistance to change could be increased if the staff felt new behaviour was expected of them without the benefit of a perceived 'luxurious' setting.

In essence, the change strategy employed followed the work of Ottoway (1976) and Lewin (1958) closely. The change agents assisted in 'unfreezing' (Lewin, 1958) established practices by working from the 'bottom-up' (Ottoway, 1976). A 'pilot site' was chosen (in this instance, one ward) to practise the new norms and style and with the joint appointees acting as on-site agents to introduce new skills and attitudes. Once the pilot site had rejected the old norms and reinforced the new, then it was ready to replicate itself within the organisation.

The individualised model of care arose eventually as a result of nurses coming together to look again at what they do; critically, sometimes cheerfully, sometimes uncomfortably. The 'coming together' may be deemed as an important feature, and much effort was needed to avoid the impression of an approach or change being imposed 'from above'. The 'bottom-up' approach requires nurses to feel they have rebuilt their own norms. The change agents (joint appointees) had to adopt a more subtle background role dropping hints or a suggestion here, mentioning a reference or a piece of research there. There was also caution in the choice of words used, with an intention to avoid language which might seem academic or distant, to minimise the potential alienating effect. Written and verbal communication about nursing practice was deliberately couched in ordinary, everyday language. Staff meetings, sometimes as often as two or three times a week, were the main method of bringing all grades together, setting up a rich and fluid exchange of ideas.

The time factor needed to produce change has been mentioned, but it is worth noting that resistance to change may take much longer to overcome in some instances than in others. In settings where patient care is the end product of activity, how much time can be allowed for new norms of behaviour to be adopted? This is one instance where industrial models of change may conflict with social ones. Taking time for change may be permissible when the end product is an inert object, but what if the outcome involves human life? What if the undesirable activity is perhaps even dangerous to the patient? A variety of leadership styles are essential. While the liberal/democratic approach was emphasised, autocratic methods were sometimes necessary, especially in the early stages, to eradicate unsound practices. Thus while some issues could await the outcome of open debate and agreement, such as a reorganisation of the patient's day, others had to be resolved instantly

CASE STUDY – *Contd*

through direct instruction, for example, the banning of routine application of Mercurochrome to pressure areas; even though this was backed up with some degree of discussion, and explanation was included.

SUMMARY

The following is a summary of the change strategies:

- Staff meetings in the formal setting at work (all grades), day and night duty.
- Multidisciplinary meetings.
- Staff meetings (single grade).
- Informal staff meetings, social events out of work hours.
- Documentation of outcome of meetings, written agreement drawn up on philosophy, attitudes, practices.
- Change agents act as enablers, facilitators 'ideas men'.
- Language choice simple, precise.
- Change 'atmosphere'; staff feel free to question, argue, debate.
- Tendency towards liberal/democratic management style, avoidance of autocracy.
- Progress reports, identification of patient/staff benefits, complimentary letters, etc., to reinforce change, encourage persistence.

Evaluation

Constant feedback also appears necessary between the change agents, the support managers, and the staff in the pilot site. It is of particular benefit if the staff can see an immediate result from their work. As Black's (1991) independent study suggests, and the many published accounts by members of staff in the unit support, it appears that enormous changes can accrue as the energies of staff are unleashed and redirected. A systematic evaluation of the effects of joint appointees as change agents has yet to emerge, but from the personal accounts a number of features appear to be common events in the pilot site over a period of time.

The points in Table 8.1 are, of course, very variable from setting to setting.

CASE STUDY – *Contd*

Table 8.1 Reported effects in the pilot site

Start ⟶ Change ⟶	After two years
Negative evaluations by learners	Positive learner evaluations
Patient turnover rate low/static with high re-admission rate	Increased patient turnover, low readmission rate
High level of complaints from patients	Low level of patient complaints
High self-discharge rate by patients	Low self-discharge rates
Few complimentary letters on care	Increased compliment rate
Higher death/transfer rate	Reduced death rate, lower transfer rate to other (e.g. long-term) care
High staff turnover	Lower staff turnover
High staff sickness/absenteeism	Lower staff sickness/absenteeism
High staff work injury	Lower staff work injury
Higher patient accident rate	Lower patient accident rate
Incidence of pressure sores raised	Reduced pressure sore incidence
Incontinence levels high	Incontinence levels reduced
Absence of systematic care planning	Care planning organised
Ritualised/routine ward activity	Patient's day personalised
Task-centred nursing	Patient-centred nursing
Difficulty recruiting staff	Easier staff recruitment
	Increased staff job-satisfaction
	Increased student success in practical assessment
	Increased teaching input
Low level of patient and staff satisfaction	Raised level of patient and staff satisfaction

In addition, the quality of nursing care is difficult to assess as so many variables are involved. For example, how far is patient turnover rate related to improvements/change in community support, medical practice, demographic changes and so on? However, a broad picture does seem to emerge when all the available information is brought together from those units where change agents have been active. They suggest a trend towards greater patient and

CASE STUDY – *Contd*

staff involvement in care, the creation of more open care systems, and a general improvement in staff and patient satisfaction. It is perhaps not insignificant or mere coincidence that such a pattern develops in settings where change agents have been involved.

Other effects

Thus far it has been possible to draw upon the experience of one particular setting where the strategies of Lewin (1958) and Ottoway (1976) had been employed. While the emphasis so far has been on changes in nursing practice, it appears from the above account that others are affected. Apart from student nurses, other staff too were drawn into a learning experience on wards which become both learner- and patient-centred. The support managers indicated that they too were affected (Black, 1991) in developing alternative styles of management with the change agents. There appears to be a trend away from autocratic, authoritarian styles of management to more open, accessible and supportive methods.

The change agents themselves appeared to adopt a more assertive style as nurses, expressing greater autonomy and advocacy in patient care, affecting relationships throughout the multidisciplinary team. Certainly the potential for conflict, especially with the established medical order (Stein, 1978), is very great when nurses indulge in the changing of practices and roles. Stein, however, in a later study (Stein *et al.*, 1990) suggests that this old relationship is slipping away as many factors such as managerial changes and the changing roles of men and women affect the way doctors and nurses perceive and work with each other.

The pilot site became a source for change in other places such as the wards of the nearby unit, other hospital wards, the division, and so on. It became a place where trained staff from other settings come for experiences to refresh their knowledge and return at some stage to their own places to act in turn as change agents. This and other manifestations demonstrate clearly how Ottoway's (1976) concept of the pilot site emerges as the new norms and style are spread to other areas following the same principles. These new sites may not be exact replicas of the pilot site, but learn from and adapt their experience to their own place of work.

In addition, a feedback system began to work. Visitors attended the ward, and members of staff (especially the change agent) became involved in external teaching activities. This led to a continuous exchange of ideas, so that constant innovation was in evidence in the open system of the pilot site (see Fig. 8.1).

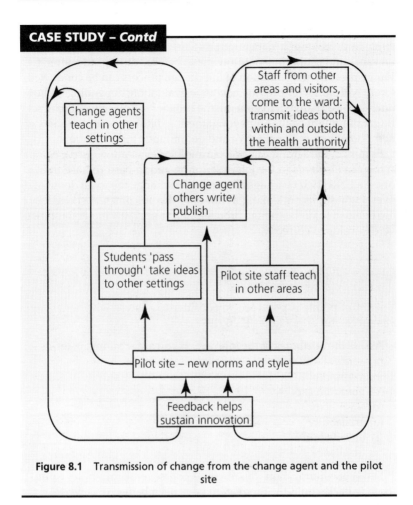

Figure 8.1 Transmission of change from the change agent and the pilot site

This case study has emphasised the role of a specifically created change agent and unit to stimulate innovation in a very institutionalised setting. However, it needs to be stressed that the principles are applicable to many settings and many roles. As has been emphasised throughout this text, all nurses are change agents whether the term is specifically embodied in their job descriptions or not. The application of the theory and process of change in the hands of the skilled change agent appears to be a significant contributor to the production of new norms in the clinical setting (Pearson, 1985; Wright, 1986; MacGuire, 1988; Black 1991).

It is also important to note that a variety of criteria had to be selected to evaluate the outcome, often profoundly affected by the nurse's own value systems (e.g. the assumption that introducing 'care planning' is a good thing). However, by identifying factors *pertinent to a particular setting* (e.g. looking at patient admission/discharge rates may not be relevant) and gathering data on these before, during and after the change process, an evaluation of the change process can be conducted. Rarely will *one* factor provide adequate evaluation, depending on how much is to be changed. In general, the broader the objectives being set, the greater might be the scope for gathering data and using a variety of methodologies both qualitative and quantitative for evaluation.

Factors in the setting can be examined for evaluation purposes, but so too can elements in the job description and in performance indicators. An ENB (1987) package has examined change theory in depth and gives suggestions on looking at not only the outcomes of change, but also evaluation of the change process itself to see if the methods shown were developed correctly.

Anatomy of an innovation

A series of points is provided to consider to analyse whether change was successful or not (after ENB, 1987):

1 Assess the attributes of the innovation you are recalling, in terms of:
   (a) relative advantage
   (b) compatibility
   (c) communicability
   (d) simplicity
   (e) trialability
   (f) observability
   (g) relevance.

Did your innovation fail on one, or several, of these counts? Looking back, could the innovation have been better conceived?

2 Assess the 'ripeness for change' of the environment into which you attempted to introduce the change. Did it show:
   (a) openness?
   (b) interpersonal and informational linkages?
   (c) freedom from organisational constraints?
   (d) supportive leadership?
   (e) trust?

If your innovation failed on one or more of these counts, there may be problems in the environment that will hinder future attempts at innovation. If you suspect this to be the case, you may find that it helps to make a more general review of organisational health. Any barriers to change, personal or organisational, that you can note will be relevant to the review.

3   Assess the 'users' of the innovation in terms of their readiness to change. What proportion (or who) are:
- innovators?
- early adopters?
- early majority?
- later majority?
- laggards?
- rejecters?

To what extent do you think users' readiness to adopt the innovation was affected by:
(a) their sense of ownership (or lack of it) of the change?
(b) their informal personal contacts (or lack of them) over the change?
(c) the involvement (or lack of it) of opinion leaders?
(d) the information and support (or lack of it) that they received in connection with the change?

4   Assess the change strategy used. Would you describe it as:
(a) rational–empirical?
(b) power–coercive?
(c) normative–re-educative?
(d) a combination?

Did you use different strategies over a period if the first one failed?

5   Assess the success of the change agent(s) involved in the innovation. How well did they carry out their functions of:
- diagnosing the problem?
- identifying and clarifying goals?
- developing appropriate strategies and tactics?
- developing good working relationships with users?

How many of the characteristics of a successful change agent did they possess?
- effort
- client orientation
- compatibility
- empathy
- use of opinion leaders
- credibility
- effort with regard to evaluation
- experience
- reflectiveness
- self-awareness
- supportiveness.

It is important, therefore, to look at change not only from the perspective of its observable results, but also at 'the living, breathing people who experience it' (Toffler, 1973).

References

Black, M. 1991 *The story of the Tameside Nursing Development Unit.* King's Fund, London.

Clark, M. 1978 Getting through the work. In: Dingwall, R. and McIntosh, J. (Eds), *Readings in the sociology of nursing.* Churchill Livingstone, Edinburgh.

Coser, R.L. 1963 Allienation and the social structure. In: Tucker, D. and Kaufert, J. (Eds), *Readings in medical sociology.* Tavistock, London.

English National Board 1987 *Managing change in nursing education: pack one: preparing for change.* ENB, London.

Friend, P. and Hayward, J. 1986 *Report of the nursing process evaluation group.* NERU Report No. 5. King's College, London.

Keyzer D.M. 1985 *Learning contracts; the trained nurse and the implementation of the nursing process.* PhD Thesis, London University.

Kitson, A.L. 1986 Indicators of quality in nursing care an alternative approach. *Journal of Advanced Nursing* **11**, 133–44.

Kuhn, T. 1970 The structure of scientific resolution. *International encyclopaedia of unified science* **2**(2), 174–86.

Lathleen, J., Bradley, S. and Smith, G. 1986 *Professional development schemes for newly registered nurses.* NERU Report No. 4. King's College, London.

Lewin, K. 1958 The group decision and social change. In: Maccoby, E. (Ed.), *Readings in social psychology.* Holt, Rinehart and Winston, London.

MacGuire, J.M. 1988 I'm your nurse, here's my card. *Nursing Times* **84** (30), 326.

McFarlane, J.K. and Castledine, G. 1982 *A guide to the practice of nursing using the nursing process.* The C.V. Mosby Co., St Louis.

Miller, E.J. and Gwynne, G.V. 1972 *A life apart.* Tavistock, London.

Orton, H. 1981 *The ward learning climate.* Royal College of Nursing, London.

Ottoway, R.M. 1976 A change strategy to implement new norms, new style and new environment in the work organisation. *Personnel Review* **5**(1), 13–15.

Parlett, M. and Hamilton, D. 1972 *Evaluation as illumination: a new approach to the study of innovatory programmes.* Occasional Paper. Centre for Research in the Education Sciences, University of Edinburgh.

Reid, E. 1986 Performance indicators. *Nursing Times* **82**(37), 448.

Rogers, C. 1969 *Freedom to learn.* Merrill, Columbus, Ohio.

Salvage, J. 1985 *The politics of nursing.* Heinemann, London.

Sheldrake, R. 1995 *Seven experiments that could change the world.* Fourth Estate, London.

Stein, L. 1978 The doctor–nurse game. In: Dingwall, R. MacIntoch. J. (Eds), *Readings in the sociology of nursing*. Churchill Livingstone, Edinburgh.

Stein, L. Watts, D.T. and Howell, M.D. 1990 The doctor–nurse game revisited. *New England Journal of Medicine* **322**, 546–549.

Toffler, A. 1973 *Future shock*. Pan Books, London.

Wells, T. 1980 *Problems in geriatric nursing*. Churchill Livingstone, Edinburgh.

Wilkinson, K.E.M.W. 1983 A blueprint for a joint appointment. *Nursing Times* **79**(42), 29–30.

Wilkinson K.E.M.W. 1984 The work in question. *Senior Nurse* **1**(28), 1720.

Wright, S.G. 1983 The best of both worlds. *Nursing Times* **79**(42), 259.

Wright, S.G. 1986 *Building and using a model of nursing*. Edward Arnold, London.

9 Conclusion: nurses and the power to change

Stephen Wright

> 'O! It is excellent to have a giant's strength, but it is tyrannous to use it like a giant.'
>
> Shakespeare, *Measure for measure*

To effect change it has so far been argued that nurses need both the knowledge and resources to do it. By virtue of sheer numbers, nurses could represent a gigantic force for social change. Even given the knowledge, would nurses *en masse* still use it? An ENB (1987) text asked, 'How effective is nursing in developing and deploying the necessary skills to take control over its own destiny? Do sufficient numbers of nurses know how 'the system' ticks, what 'power' is and how to use it, and how to function as change agents?'

Knowledge of change would not only equip nurses to be better change agents, it would also help them (knowing why, how and where it is coming from) to resist change when appropriate. Resistance to change is not always a negative process, even if it might annoy those seeking to change things, because it 'fires the proponents of change to justify and promote the reasons for their proposals' (ENB, 1987). After all, change is not always for the better, and resistance is sometimes well-founded, given the pitfalls in nursing history.

Teaching nurses how to be change agents rarely finds its way into the curriculum of schools of nursing. True, some argument might, with some justification, be put forward that there is little time to squeeze it in among other, apparently more pressing, needs. However, might there not also be some reluctance on the part of those in power to include this subject? The established system of health care, might at the very least, be rocked to its foundations. There are 500 000 nurses in the UK. Just imagine the effect, not only on nursing in the health service, but in society as a whole, if such a vast army of skilled change agents was unleashed upon them!

Meanwhile, nursing is held in check. As a female-dominated occupation, it is still inhibited in its potential in a society which still largely functions and sets priorities around male values, although there are many signs as suggested in previous chapters that this *status quo* is shifting. The discipline is still affected to some degree by the pervasive (male) medical model which prefers to keep nurses in their place. Attempts to rectify this imbalance continue, whether it be through the professional lobbying, persuasion and evidence being produced by organisations such as the RCN and other unions and groups of nurses, the efforts to create more leadership and MBA programmes for nurses or the accumulating body of nursing research which attests to its effectiveness. All these factors and more, such as the changing roles of doctors and nurses, the expansion of nursing roles, changing public perceptions and expectations and changes to the way health care is organised, are creating a rich and volatile climate in which change is under way. The future of nursing is inextricably linked also with the changing role of women. How women shift their place in the world and their view of themselves will have a knock-on effect in nursing, which continues to employ them in very large numbers (about 90% of the workforce). More men in nursing, who are still particularly advantaged in gaining the most senior positions, the shift in the power structures between nurses and doctors, and the new health service managers are all factors adding more complexity and catalysts for change to the equation. Change in nursing is coming, but often painfully slowly in a system which still adheres to hierarchical, bureaucratic values espousing obedience, routine and authority in many areas.

To move away from this is not to advocate anarchy, but to wean nursing away from the 'narcissistic mirror offered by medicine' (Oakley, 1984) so that it occupies its rightful place in the chorus of health care. Moving nursing into a position where it would dominate all other professions would be as unhelpful to those it serves – the patients or clients – as is nursing's currently oppressed status. Professional power tends to corrupt into a 'conspiracy against the laity' (Freidson, 1970). The professional power to change things, which this book has espoused, seeks not mastery but partnership; with clients and other disciplines. In this sense, nursing cannot, and must not, adhere to the traditional sociological definition of a profession. If nursing does this, it may become like the pigs in *Animal farm* (Orwell, 1951), 'Twelve voices were shouting in anger, and they were all alike. No question, now, what had happened to the faces of the pigs. The creatures outside looked from pig to man, and from man to pig, and from pig to man again; but already it was impossible to say which was which'.

At the same time, seeing nursing as in conflict with management, other professions, and with clients is an outmoded paradigm. It is helpful to no one to see the position of nurses simply as the result of dominance by others. The picture is far more complex, far more subtle.

Nursing, after all, is still quite young, as professions go, with enormous potential for the future.

At this stage, it would be useful to reconsider some of the salient points as to the ways in which nurses can become effective change agents.

- *Acquire knowledge.* Attend a course or conference, read widely, take out a learning contract with a teacher or mentor, develop a clinical supervision and reflective practice relationship, start work on a distance learning package, learn about change theory. Get to know more about how you and the organisation tick. Take a course in self-awareness and assertiveness. Awareness of your own situation is the first step on the road to changing the world around you.

- *Learn who the key people are in your organisation and how to lobby them for support.* Get them to sign up to the changes you are proposing so that you are not left high and dry on your own if something goes wrong. (The early King's Fund NDU programme required, for example, the chief executive of the employing organisation to sign a letter of support for the changes.)

- *Own the process of change.* Work with colleagues in small or large groups. Set up a quality circle, standard-setting group or similar, for example, to determine for yourself the things you would like to change. Work out an action plan for change, helping to share the vision, specifying who is responsible for what, and involving as many colleagues as possible. Is a clinical leader needed to guide everyone? Does someone have to be identified to champion the changes? Develop an inclusive rather than exclusive approach to change with your colleagues – even if they reject what you are doing, always keep the door open for interest and participation.

- *Set out your goals clearly so that you have your vision for a better future always before you and map out how you wish to achieve them.* Stay with things that you care about, those that have heart and meaning for you; this helps to sustain your commitment and keep you on a path that feels right and authentic to you. Question why change is proposed, who will benefit from it, and whether it is acceptable to you and your colleagues both morally and ethically.

- *Learn about, select and use a change strategy or perhaps elements of more than one which work for you, such as those described in the early chapters of this book.* What is the best position to be in to effect change? What can you do where you are now? Assess, plan, implement and evaluate.

- *Look after yourself.* Check that what you wish to do lies within the framework of your accountability. Take time for yourself. Nothing is so important that it burns you out, drains you completely, or destroys your valued relationships.

- *Give it time.* Changing the organisation of even one ward or one small unit can take years. Don't be disappointed if it isn't all perfect overnight.
- *Form a conspiracy.* Get colleagues, managers, teachers, on your side. Work slowly, deliberately through the power of the group to achieve your goals. Act at both a personal and political level.
- *Identify ways of gaining peer support.* Do this by networking, shadowing, joining a learning set, attending a course, conference or similar interest group. Consider creating a support network if a suitable one does not already exist for you.
- *Commit yourself to your responsibilities and to the change process, but do not forget to take care of yourself and your colleagues.* There is life beyond nursing. Create and enjoy social events and cultivate a wide circle of friends and interests – especially outside nursing.
- *Accept that change is evolutionary; be prepared for holdups, setbacks.* Be flexible, prepared to adapt your strategy, think again, change course.
- *Don't feel guilty if it doesn't all go right.* It isn't all your fault. Look back upon what you have done well, value it, cherish it, and do this on a regular basis so the progress you have made, however small, is not lost sight of. There may be mountains ahead, but many hills lie behind that you have already climbed.
- *Set your sights within your range.* Aim for things which you know you *can* do. Start small and work up to the big goals, achieving each step as you go and avoiding disappointment.
- *Check up on your own skills.* Becoming a change agent is a lifelong process. Engage others as you go along. Develop your communication skills. Give praise to colleagues rather than criticism.
- *Don't underestimate the qualities you need to change things.* Combine your own drive with physical and psychological stamina. Keeping yourself physically fit is often as important as looking after your personal and professional relationships.
- *Keep up to date and help colleagues to do the same.* Disseminate your ideas using your colleagues. Provide books, journals, written information, so that those involved in the change process can become as enlightened as you are!
- *Focus on one place at a time.* Set up a pilot site and use it as the base to achieve your aims. This can itself become a transmission site for new ideas (see Chapter 6).
- *Plan an evaluation strategy for before, during, and after the change process.* Evaluation should be completed before a change is transmitted to other sites. This will help justify your case, and can give you and your colleagues the evidence for achievement.
- *Document what you do.* Write about it and let others know about it. Consider it for publication, others can learn from your experience.

- *Become political, both with a big and small 'p'.* It is not only important to influence your own organisation but to influence others in power too. Next time the politicians call, ask them what they propose to do about your difficulties. If nurses become 'involved in and participate in political decision-making through the nursing organisations and in the political parties, I believe they will be an unstoppable force for change' (Clay, 1987).
- *Map out your own career.* Seek careers advice. Get yourself into a position of power best suited to effect the kind of changes you want.
- *Explore your values, clarify your ideals;* they are a real source of strength in difficult times.

To be a change agent is a difficult task, but it provides a path full of challenge, opportunities and possibilities – they are the things which make us human. As a change agent, the nurse has to draw upon all the resources of physical and psychological stamina; this may test your credibility to its limits, along with your powers of intellect and communication. Subtlety, guile, imagination, empathy, resourcefulness: these are the tools, the stock in trade of those who would change things, creating a climate of change not only among small groups of colleagues, but ultimately to a change culture that exists at all levels of the organisation. The organisation can develop a culture of learning and change, where change is a way of life and changes become less threatening, part of the architecture of the setting. Often the organisation is strong and repressive, and in such places it takes courage and commitment to hold onto our values and continue working when we know things could be different. Being bicultural, working in a place where things are not right but staying there and working quietly to bring them to your own view takes strength and staying power, and an ability to set your limits and care for yourself. At other times, however, an organisation can be ripe for change as, for example, when new government policies destabilise existing systems and provide an expectation of change. Nurses have to be ready to move in when the ideal opportunity arrives; when they do not, others are only too ready and willing to fill the vacuum.

There are many possible methods of attempting change in nursing. With its hierarchical system of organisation, its immense size in terms of numbers, and its place in the establishment under the umbrella of health care, it is perhaps one of the most difficult areas to innovate, especially where established attitudes and practices are challenged. Yet it is precisely these reasons which can contribute to nursing's strength in the potential for change.

It may be argued that success, where it is achieved, is due in no small measure to those change agents with the courage and energy to commit themselves to change, and to those who support them. When nurses get together we often seem to spend much time claiming that everything is awful, or telling ourselves how wonderful we are. Neither pattern serves us or our patients well, and little changes as a result. Learning to be a change agent empowers us to move out of such patterns that keep us stuck in ways that do not help us. This book has attempted to explore ways of implementing change in a planned and systematic way, and with a sound theoretical base. Combined with the personal and intuitive powers of each nurse, change is a powerful force. It is contended that, although the style and emphasis of the change method may differ, change must be organised in this way if it is to attain its goal of infusing new norms and practices into the system. Unplanned and disordered change may lead to dissipation and wastage of much energy at great personal cost. The price of change where this occurs may be considered unacceptable. When nurses take on their role as change agents, then change in nursing practice is achievable. In this way, innovative, creative and personalised nursing can emerge when those features which are changed become an accepted part of the new order. We owe it to ourselves. We owe it to our patients. Nurses can do it.

References

Clay, T. 1987 *Nurses, power and politics.* Heinemann, London.
English National Board 1987 *Managing change in nursing education. Pack One: Preparing for change.* ENB, London.
Freidson, E. 1970 *The profession of medicine.* Dodd Mead, New York.
Oakley, A. 1984 The importance of being a nurse. *Nursing Times* **12**, 246.
Orwell, G. 1951 *Animal farm.* Penguin, Harmondsworth.

Index

Page numbers printed in **bold** type refer to figures; those in *italic* to tables